OXFORD MEDICAL PUBLICA

A Basic Formulary for General Practice

PRACTICAL GUIDES FOR GENERAL PRACTICE

Editorial Board

J. A. Muir Gray, Community Physician,
Oxfordshire Health Authority.
Ann McPherson, General Practitioner, Oxford.
Michael Bull, GP Tutor, Oxford.
John Tasker, GP Tutor, North Oxfordshire.

1. *Cervical screening: a practical guide*
   Ann McPherson
3. *Radiology*
   Robert F. Bury
4. *Stroke*
   Derick Wade
5. *Alcohol*
   P. Anderson
6. *Breast cancer screening*
   Joan Austoker and John Humphreys
7. *Computers: a guide to choosing and using*
   Tom Stewart and Andrew Willis
8. *Immunizing children*
   Sue Sefi and J. A. Macfarlane
9. *On-call: out of hours telephone calls and home visits*
   James D. E. Knox
10. *Breast cancer screening* (Scottish edition)
    Joan Austoker and John Humphreys (with M. Maureen Roberts)
11. *Screening tests used in pre-school child surveillance*
    J. A. Macfarlane and Sue Sefi
12. *A basic formulary for general practice* (second edition)
    G. B. Grant, D. A. Gregory, and T. D. van Zwanenberg

Forthcoming

Non-insulin-dependent diabetes
Ann-Louise Kinmonth

A Basic Formulary for General Practice

Practical Guides for General Practice 12

Second Edition

G. B. GRANT, D. A. GREGORY, and
T. D. van ZWANENBERG

*Division of Primary Health Care,
University of Newcastle upon Tyne*

Oxford Melbourne Toronto
OXFORD UNIVERSITY PRESS
1990

Oxford University Press, Walton Street, Oxford OX2 6DP
Oxford New York Toronto
Delhi Bombay Calcutta Madras Karachi
Petaling Jaya Singapore Hong Kong Tokyo
Nairobi Dar es Salaam Cape Town
Melbourne Auckland

and associated companies in
Berlin Ibadan

Oxford is a trade mark of Oxford University Press

Published in the United States
by Oxford University Press, New York

© G. B. Grant, D. A. Gregory, and T. D. van Zwanenberg, 1990

All rights reserved. No part of this publication may be reproduced,
stored in a retrieval system, or transmitted, in any form or by any means,
electronic, mechanical, photocopying, recording, or otherwise, without
the prior permission of Oxford University Press.

This book is sold subject to the condition that it shall not, by way
of trade or otherwise, be lent, re-sold, hired out, or otherwise circulated
without the publisher's prior consent in any form of binding or cover
other than that in which it is published and without a similar condition
including this condition being imposed on the subsequent purchaser.

British Library Cataloguing in Publication Data
Grant, G. B. (George Bryce)
A basic formulary for general practice.—2nd ed.
1. Medicine. Drug therapy
I. Title   II. Gregory, D. A. (David Andrew)   III. van
Zwanenberg, T. D.   IV. Series
615.58
ISBN 0-19-261951-9

Library of Congress Cataloging in Publication Data
Grant, G. B. (George Bryce)
A basic formulary for general practice/G. B. Grant, D. A. Gregory,
and T. D. van Zwanenberg.—2nd ed.
p. cm.—(Practical guides for general practice; 12)
(Oxford medical publications)
1. Chemotherapy—Handbooks, manuals, etc. 2. Family medicine—
Handbooks, manuals, etc.   I. Gregory, D. A. (David Andrew)
II. van Zwanenberg, T. D.   III. Title.   IV. Series.   V. Series:
Oxford medical publications.
[DNLM: 1. Drug therapy—handbooks.   2. Formularies—Great Britain—
handbooks. W1 PR141NK no. 12/QV 39 G7616b]
RM262.G69   1990   615.5'8—dc20   90-7007
ISBN 0-19-261951-9

Set by Cotswold Typesetting Ltd, Cheltenham
Printed in Great Britain by Dotesios Printers Ltd., Trowbridge, Wilts.

Foreword

Prescribing drugs is one of the most important, and certainly the most expensive, professional activity that general practitioners undertake. The rational use of drugs demands that doctors prescribe effectively, safely, and economically. By international standards, prescribing in the United Kingdom is not excessive. Thus, the average member of the British public receives 7 prescriptions per annum, compared to the 16 given each year to Americans. Yet the task of making sensible choices from the wide variety of available products is daunting; and experience has shown that general practitioners can deliver the highest standards of medical care to their patients with a relatively small range of medicines.

The first edition of this formulary, designed specifically for the needs of general practitioners, drew on the experience of those general practitioners who teach medical students at the University of Newcastle upon Tyne. It provided information on when *not* to use drugs as well as offering sensible, down-to-earth advice on both the selection and care of specific agents. It has been a useful introduction to the real world for medical students during their general practice attachments and an invaluable primer for general practice trainees. It has been of substantial value to established practitioners to the extent that several FPCs provided copies for all their doctors. And it has had an international impact: for, by sheer coincidence, its close resemblance to the WHO's Model List of Essential Drugs has underpinned the efforts of primary health care planners in many developed, and developing, countries to encourage rational drug usage.

The second edition continues the tradition of the first. It has been revised in the light of discussions with Tyneside general practitioners, to take acount of changes in clinical practice and increased understanding of drug action. The format remains unchanged and I am sure that this edition will make an even greater contribution to primary health care than its predecessor.

Michael D. Rawlins
Professor of Clinical Pharmacology,
University of Newcastle upon Tyne

Preface to the First Edition

This formulary was developed in order to provide simple and appropriate treatment for 90 per cent of the conditions presenting in general practice.

We compiled it in association with about twenty general practitioners who are Clinical Tutors to medical students at Newcastle University. These general practitioners came from different practices, and in a series of meetings (including a residential weekend) we modified and added to the formulary until a consensus was reached.

Advice of two consultant colleagues was obtained on specific matters.

The formulary is presented as an alphabetical list of conditions with the appropriate drug treatment, including dosage and price (cost, though important, was not regarded as the major consideration).

Except for a few proprietary combination preparations (e.g. oral contraceptives) we have used only generic names of drugs. In general, and only where there was strong evidence of a drug's superiority over other treatment, we have not included drugs which have been in use for less than five years.

We excluded most drugs which are used only in emergencies. Drugs normally initiated in a hospital are listed only in the appendix.

The list of conditions reflects the broad therapeutic areas seen in general practice, so that some conditions will be an actual diagnosis (e.g. asthma) and others will be symptoms (e.g. pain).

The more common skin conditions are also included.

We have specified what we think are the most appropriate drugs for each condition and have not normally included several drugs with identical actions. Where a choice of drugs is given, we have placed them in what we consider a sensible order. We have also set out some notes about diagnosis and the drugs. These notes are in no way meant to be comprehensive.

We know by controlled testing in several diverse practices that by using this formulary a general practitioner can prescribe for about 90 per cent of conditions encountered and which require a drug. This leaves the practitioner free to prescribe other drugs in special circumstances (e.g. drug-sensitivity, renal and hepatic disease).

We have also used this formulary in teaching medical students and they have found it of value.

It is easier and safer to become familiar with the action, side-effects, contra-indications, and drug interactions of a limited number of well-proven preparations. We believe that a general practitioner using this formulary will be able to prescribe rationally, safely, and cheaply.

We hope you will find this pocket formulary of great use to you in your practice. We intend to revise the formulary at regular intervals, and would welcome suggestions and comments from readers.

Newcastle upon Tyne G. B. G.
1986 D. A. G.
  T. D. v. Z.

Preface to the Second Edition

Soon after the publication of the first edition it became obvious that revision would be necessary in order to represent the current prescribing of the authors and their colleagues. We have again followed the method we used in compiling the first edition.[1]

Meetings with all the undergraduate tutors in general practice in Newcastle took place to debate the changes necessary. The proposed amendments were tested in more than 5000 consultations by this group, and these are reflected in the text.

The present method of pricing prescriptions for payment to pharmacy contractors differs from that in operation in 1986. This section has been rewritten by Mr. L. S. Ray, MPS.

The size and format of the book had been well received by colleagues in the United Kingdom and Europe. The format has therefore not been altered, but we have added a section on prescribing in terminal care.

We hope readers will find this edition informative and easy to use. We would again welcome comments.

Newcastle upon Tyne   G. B. G.
1989   D. A. G.
                                                                                          T. D. v. Z.

---

[1]Grant, G. B., Gregory, D. A., and van Zwanenberg, T. D. (1985). Development of a limited formulary for General Practice, *Lancet* i, 1030-1.

Acknowledgements

The authors would like to thank those many people who have assisted with the compilation and revision of this formulary, without whose help it would not have been possible.

Over twenty general practitioners collaborated by recording their prescribing, and after a series of meetings were able to reach a consensus on rational prescribing in general practice. This we believe makes the formulary a valid one and we would like to thank them most sincerely.

We received sound advice and constructive criticism from Emeritus Professor J. H. Walker and Professor M. D. Rawlins which greatly encouraged us in our efforts. We also received expert advice from Dr. S. Comaish, dermatology; Dr. C. Edwards, antibiotics; Mr. P. Hopley, pharmaceuticals; Mr. L. Ray, pricing prescriptions; Dr. C. Regnard, terminal care; and Mr. E. Thomas, hormone replacement therapy. Anne Prasad, Executive Editor of the British National Formulary, gave us a great deal of constructive help especially in relation to dosage.

Finally, without the skill, patience, and long hours of work of Mrs Karen Cowley and Miss Anne Corradine with the first edition, and Mrs Linda Redpath with the second, the formulary would never have been completed.

Proprietary drugs

Most of the drugs in the formulary are generic. However, some proprietary combination preparations are included:

All oral contraceptives
Alphosyl
Anusol
Anusol-HC
Asilone
Betadine
Cyclo-progynova
Dioralyte
Dithrocream
Dyazide
Gaviscon
Locorten-vioform
Maalox
Madopar
Nuelin
Nystaform-HC
Otosporin
Polytar
Premarin
Pripsen
Sinemet

Contents

List of abbreviations	xv
Costing prescriptions	xvi
Allergy	1
Hayfever, urticaria	1
Anaemia	2
Angina pectoris	4
Anxiety/agitation	6
Anxiety	6
Agitation	6
Arthritis	7
Gout	8
Asthma	9
Bronchitis	12
Cardiac failure	14
Constipation	16
Contraception	18
Depression	20
Diarrhoea and inflammatory bowel disease	22
Dyspepsia, oesophagitis, and peptic ulcer	24
Endocrine conditions	26
Diabetes mellitus (non-insulin dependent)	26
Hypothyroidism	27
Eye conditions	28
Blepharitis/conjunctivitis	28
Dry eyes	28
Dendritic corneal ulcer	28

Hypertension	29
Insomnia	32
Irritable bowel syndrome	33
Anal discomfort	34
Menopause	35
Migraine	36
Mouth infections	38
Mouth ulcers	38
Oral candidiasis	39
Herpetic stomatitis/Herpes labialis	39
Oral hygiene	40
Dental abscess	40
Nausea and/or vomiting and/or vertigo	41
Neurological disorders	42
Epilepsy	42
Neuralgia	43
Spasticity	43
Parkinsonism	44
Otitis externa	45
Ear wax	46
Pain	46
Night cramps	48
Premenstrual syndrome	49
Dysmenorrhoea	49
Pruritus vulvae/vaginal discharge	50
Skin conditions	52
Acute eczema/Dermatitis	52
Dry eczema/Ichthyosis	52
Nappy rash	52
Psoriasis	52
Skin infections	54
Impetigo	54
Cellulitis	54
Erysipelas	55
Acne vulgaris	55

Furunculosis	56
Scabies	56
Tinea	57
Herpes simplex	57
Herpes zoster	57
Warts	57
Terminal care—symptom control	59
Pain	59
Nausea and vomiting	59
Constipation and diarrhoea	60
Anorexia	61
Restlessness and confusion	61
Raised intracranial pressure	61
Dry mouth/Fungal infection	61
Respiratory symptoms	62
Upper respiratory tract infections	63
The common cold	63
Catarrh	63
Cough	64
Sinusitis	64
Throat infections	65
Otitis media	66
Urinary tract conditions	68
Acute infection	68
Enuresis	69
Detrusor instability	69
Worms	70
Appendix: Drug treatments normally initiated by hospital consultants	71
Index	75

Abbreviations

ACE	angiotensin-converting enzyme
AIDS	acquired immunodeficiency syndrome
amps	ampoules
BNF	*British National Formulary*
BP	*British Pharmacopoeia*
caps	capsules
CNS	central nervous system
CSM	Committee for the Safety of Medicines
CXR	chest X-ray
e.c.	enteric-coated
ECG	electrocardiograph
ESR	erythrocyte sedimentation rate
g	grams
Hb	haemoglobin
HIV	human immunodeficiency virus
HRT	hormone replacement therapy
i.v.	intravenous
kg	kilogram
MAOI	monoamine oxidase inhibitors
mg	milligram
ml	millilitre
MSU	mid-stream urine specimen
NSAID	non-steroidal anti-inflammatory drug
OTC	over the counter
s.r.	slow-release
suppos	suppositories
tabs	tablets
TSH	thyroid stimulating hormone
UTI	urinary tract infection
WBC	white blood count

Costing prescriptions

The cost of drugs (as at September 1989) is usually stated as the cost of 100 tablets, capsules, or 500 ml of a liquid. The current cost of drugs can be updated from the most recent edition of the *British National Formulary.* The actual cost to the National Health Service of any particular prescription, based on the payments made to a pharmacy dispensing 3000 scripts a month, may be calculated from the following formula.

Formula	*Example* 28 capsules Ampicillin 250 mg
Cost of ingredients	93.4p
On-cost of 5%	4.6p
Less discount of 8%	−7.4p
Container @ 3.8p	3.8p
Dispensing fee 95.3p	95.3p
	189.7p

It should be noted that there are no additional payments for rent, rates, or ancillary staff, the cost of which are borne by the contractor.

The proposal to make original pack dispensing mandatory, should, providing standardized packs can be agreed, make prescribing and dispensing simpler, safer, and more economical.

Allergy

Hayfever, Urticaria

Treatment

Chlorpheniramine OTC	Adult dose:	4 mg three times daily.
	Child dose:	Under 1 year: 1 mg twice daily; 1-5 years: 1-2 mg three times daily; 6-12 years: 2-4 mg three times daily.
Terfenadine OTC	Adult dose:	60 mg twice daily.
	Child dose:	30 mg twice daily (not recommended under 6 years of age).
Beclomethasone (nasal spray)	Adult and child dose:	50 micrograms to each nostril up to four times daily (not recommended under 6 years of age).

Prophylaxis

Sodium cromoglycate	Adult and child dose:	20 mg by nasal insufflation four times daily; or 2 per cent nasal spray four times daily (not recommended for children under 6 years); and/or 2 per cent eye drops four times daily.

Important notes

1. Chlorpheniramine, which is usually sedative, and terfenadine, which is rarely so, are alternative antihistamines. Either may be used in combination with beclomethasone spray and/or sodium cromoglycate.
2. Chlorpheniramine may potentiate the effects of alcohol and sedative CNS drugs. It may also cause other anticholinergic side-effects.
3. As sedation is possible, patients should be warned if driving or operating machinery.
4. Desensitizing injections are of doubtful benefit and should not be used in general practice.

Cost

Chlorpheniramine	4 mg	100 tabs	=	90p
	2 mg/5 ml syrup	500 ml	=	97p
Terfenadine	60 mg	100 tabs	=	£9.67
	30 mg/5 ml suspension	500 ml	=	£10.60
Beclomethasone	Nasal spray	200 doses	=	£5.01
Sodium cromoglycate	2% eye drops	13.5 ml	=	£5.59
	2% metered nasal spray	26 ml	=	£5.36
	10 mg cartridge	100 caps	=	£3.89

Anaemia

Treatment

Iron deficiency
Ferrous sulphate
OTC

Adult dose: 200 mg three times daily.

Child dose: Under 1 year: 60 mg three times daily;
1–5 years: 120 mg three times daily;
6–12 years: 200 mg three times daily.

Ferrous gluconate
OTC
Adult dose: 300 mg twice daily.

Vitamin B$_{12}$ deficiency
Hydroxocobalamin
Adult and child dose: Initially: 1 mg repeated 5 times at intervals of 2–3 days; maintenance: 1 mg every 3 months.

Folic acid deficiency
Folic acid
Adult dose: Initially: 15 mg daily for 14 days; maintenance: 5 mg every 1–7 days.

Important notes

1. Proper diagnosis is essential.
2. Combined iron/folic acid preparations contain very little folic acid.
3. Iron deficiency anaemia in the elderly may be caused by long term use of NSAIDs or large bowel malignancy.
4. Iron salts can cause gastrointestinal side-effects: nausea, epigastric pain, diarrhoea, or constipation.
5. Antacids and tetracyclines can cause reduced therapeutic response to iron preparations.

Cost

Ferrous sulphate	200 mg	100 tabs =	35p
	60 mg/5 ml mixture	500 ml =	45p
Ferrous gluconate	300 mg	100 tabs =	60p
Hydroxocobalamin	250 micrograms	5 amps =	45p
	1000 micrograms	5 amps =	90p
Folic acid	5 mg	100 tabs =	30p

Angina pectoris

Treatment

Short-acting nitrates
Glyceryl trinitrate OTC Adult dose: 500 microgram tablet or 400 microgram aerosol spray sublingually as required.

Long-acting nitrates
Isosorbide dinitrate OTC Adult dose: 10–40 mg three times daily.
or
Isosorbide mononitrate Adult dose: 10–40 mg twice or three times daily.

Beta-blockers
Propranolol Adult dose: 40–160 mg twice daily.
or
Atenolol Adult dose: 50–100 mg daily.
or
Metoprolol Adult dose: 50–200 mg daily in one or two doses.

Calcium antagonists
Nifedipine Adult dose: 5–20 mg three times daily.

Important notes

1. Treat predisposing causes: smoking, hypertension, obesity, anaemia, arrhythmias, etc.
2. Basic investigations: CXR; ECG; Hb; TSH; urinalysis.
3. Glyceryl trinitrate tablets deteriorate and should not be used 8 weeks after opening. The bottle should not contain cotton wool. Some patients find the aerosol spray more convenient, and it remains effective for up to 2 years.

4. Nitrates can cause flushing, headache, tachycardia, and syncope. The theoretical advantage of isosorbide mononitrate over dinitrate has yet to be demonstrated in practice. Tolerance to nitrates may occur.

5. Beta-blockers can cause bradycardia, heart failure, bronchospasm, peripheral vasoconstriction, gastrointestinal disturbances, vivid dreams, insomnia, and fatigue. They should not be used in asthma, heart failure, or heart block, and may aggravate intermittent claudication.

6. Nifedipine should be withdrawn if angina worsens shortly after starting therapy. Nifedipine capsules 5 mg or 10 mg may be chewed for immediate relief. A sustained release preparation of 10 mg or 20 mg is also available.

7. Nifedipine side-effects are similar to those of nitrates.

8. Aspirin in the dosage of 75 mg daily or 300 mg on alternate days is appropriate preventive treatment following myocardial infarction, or in unstable angina.

Cost

Glyceryl trinitrate	500 micrograms	100 tabs =	44p
	400 micrograms metered aerosol	200 doses =	£3.36
Isosorbide dinitrate	10 mg	100 tabs =	£1.00
	20 mg	100 tabs =	£2.00
	30 mg	100 tabs =	£2.56
Isosorbide mononitrate	10 mg	100 tabs =	£5.80
	20 mg	100 tabs =	£8.00
	40 mg	100 tabs =	£13.95
Propranolol	10 mg	100 tabs =	25p
	40 mg	100 tabs =	40p
	80 mg	100 tabs =	75p
	160 mg s.r.	100 tabs =	£1.30
Atenolol	50 mg	100 tabs =	£16.89
	100 mg	100 tabs =	£23.86
Metoprolol	50 mg	100 tabs =	£4.70
	100 mg	100 tabs =	£8.75
Nifedipine	5 mg	100 caps =	£7.90
	10 mg	100 caps =	£10.10
	10 mg s.r.	100 tabs =	£14.89
	20 mg s.r.	100 tabs =	£19.30

Anxiety/Agitation

Anxiety

Treatment

Propranolol	Adult dose:	10–40 mg twice or three times daily.
Diazepam	Adult dose:	2–10 mg twice or three times daily.

Important notes

1. Worry is not an illness, nor is unhappiness.
2. Anxiety may be the presenting symptom of a depressive illness, which should not be treated with a benzodiazepine.
3. Benzodiazepine therapy of any kind can cause long-term dependence with subsequent withdrawal symptoms, and should therefore only be prescribed for a very short time.
4. Propranolol may be an effective treatment for the somatic symptoms of anxiety. For propranolol side-effects, *see under* beta-blockers, in Angina section.
5. Benzodiazepines can cause nausea, constipation, drowsiness, dizziness, ataxia, confusion (especially in the elderly), depression, and occasionally rashes and blood dyscrasias.
6. Lorazepam is addictive and should not be used. Withdrawal should be undertaken with great care under diazepam cover.

Agitation

Treatment

Chlorpromazine	Adult dose:	10–100 mg three or four times daily.
	Child dose:	Up to 5 years: 5–10 mg three times daily; 6–12 years: $\frac{1}{2}$–$\frac{1}{3}$ adult dose.
Thioridazine	Adult dose:	25–100 mg three times daily.

Important notes

1. Agitation is a common problem in the elderly. Proper diagnosis is essential, as it may be the presenting symptom of serious organic disease, depression, or dementia.
2. Extrapyramidal effects may occur with the major tranquillizers. These may be dose-related, related to the actual drug, or be due to patient idiosyncrasy.
3. Common side-effects include dry mouth, constipation, hypotension (particularly in the elderly), drowsiness, paradoxical agitation, depression, Parkinsonism, tardive dyskinesia, and urinary retention.

Cost

Propranolol	10 mg	100 tabs = 25p
	40 mg	100 tabs = 40p
Diazepam	2 mg	100 tabs = 10p
	5 mg	100 tabs = 13p
Chlorpromazine	10 mg	100 tabs = 55p
	25 mg	100 tabs = 75p
	50 mg	100 tabs = £1.65
	100 mg	100 tabs = £3.10
	25 mg/5 ml syrup	500 ml = £1.30
	25 mg/5 ml injection	10 amps = £2.70
Thioridazine	10 mg	100 tabs = £1.15
	25 mg	100 tabs = £1.60
	50 mg	100 tabs = £3.05
	100 mg	100 tabs = £5.80

Arthritis

Treatment

Ibuprofen OTC	Adult dose:	200–600 mg four times daily.
	Child dose:	20 mg/kg weight daily, in divided doses.

Naproxen	Adult dose:	250–500 mg twice daily.
Piroxicam	Adult dose:	20 mg daily.
Indomethacin	Adult dose:	25–50 mg four times daily. *Rectally:* 100 mg twice daily.
Methylprednisolone acetate injection		4–80 mg according to site of lesion.

Important notes

1. All non-steroidal anti-inflammatory drugs may cause nausea, vomiting, peptic ulceration, anaemia from occult blood loss, and haematemesis/melaena.

2. Aspirin which patients may purchase OTC may also cause tinnitus, deafness, urticaria, angioneurotic oedema, and bronchospasm.

3. Ibuprofen causes less side-effects than other NSAIDs and may be purchased OTC under a variety of proprietary names.

4. NSAIDs can also cause tinnitus, blurred vision, bronchospasm, depression, confusion, insomnia, peripheral neuropathy, convulsions, psychiatric disturbances, rashes, and blood dyscrasias.

5. Analgesics, other NSAIDs and suppressive drugs may be required, if the arthritis does not respond.

6. Methylprednisolone local injection with lignocaine may be used for soft tissue lesions such as tennis elbow or for intra-articular injections.

Gout

Treatment

Indomethacin or	Adult dose:	50 mg four times daily.
Naproxen	Adult dose:	500–750 mg twice daily.

Prophylaxis

Allopurinol	Adult dose:	100–900 mg daily.

Important notes

1. Check serum uric acid before prophylactic treatment.
2. Concurrent indomethacin/naproxen advisable initially with allopurinol.
3. Allopurinol may cause gastrointestinal irritation and rashes.

Cost

Ibuprofen	200 mg	100 tabs	= £1.30
	400 mg	100 tabs	= £2.55
	600 mg	100 tabs	= £6.80
	100 mg/5 ml syrup	500 ml	= £3.85
Naproxen	250 mg	100 tabs	= £8.20
	500 mg	100 tabs	= £16.40
	500 mg suppos	30 suppos	= £8.70
Piroxicam	10 mg	100 tabs	= £14.25
	20 mg	100 tabs	= £18.85
Indomethacin	25 mg	100 tabs	= 90p
	50 mg	100 tabs	= £2.75
	100 mg suppos	30 suppos	= £5.49
Allopurinol	100 mg	100 tabs	= £2.50
	300 mg	100 tabs	= £13.50
Methylprednisolone	40 mg/ml injection	1 amp	= £2.59
Lignocaine 1%	2 ml injection	1 amp	= 5p

Asthma

Treatment

Salbutamol	Adult dose:	*Oral:* 1–8 mg four times daily. *Inhaled:* 100–800 micrograms every 4–6 hours.

10 Asthma

	Child dose:	*Oral:* 2-5 years: 1-2 mg four times daily; 6-12 years: 2 mg four times daily. *Inhaled:* 100 micrograms four times daily.
Terbutaline	Adult dose:	*Oral:* 5 mg two to three times daily. *Inhaled:* 250-500 micrograms every 4 hours as necessary.
	Child dose:	*Oral:* 3-6 years: 0.75-1.5 mg three times daily; 7-12 years: 2.5 mg two to three times daily. *Inhaled:* up to 100 micrograms every 4 hours as necessary.
Theophylline s.r. OTC	Adult dose: Child dose:	175-500 mg twice daily. 175 mg every 12 hours (over 6 years of age).
Prednisolone	Adult dose:	1-20 mg four times daily.
Beclomethasone	Adult dose:	*Inhaled:* 100-500 micrograms four times daily.
	Child dose:	50-100 micrograms four times daily.

Prophylaxis

Sodium cromoglycate	Adult and child dose:	*Inhaled:* 5 mg four times daily (aerosol) or 20 mg four times daily (insufflation).

Important notes

1. Advise the patient to stop smoking. Exclude possible extrinsic causative factors.

2. Salbutamol may cause palpitations, hypotension, tremor, and headaches. It should be used with caution in hyperthyroidism, ischaemic heart disease, hypertension, pregnancy, and elderly patients.

3. Check serum theophylline concentration is within therapeutic range. The correct level is critical. Prescribers are advised to specify proprietary preparation, as bio-availability varies. Caution: concomitant administration of i.v. aminophylline – particular care in elderly patients.

4. Theophylline may cause nausea, vomiting, vertigo, insomnia, confusion, and convulsions.

5. Corticosteroids including prednisolone have many serious side-effects with long-term use, the most important of which are: peptic ulceration, hypertension, fluid retention, cataracts, diabetes, osteoporosis (especially in the elderly), mental disturbances, Cushing's syndrome, exacerbation of infections, and adrenal suppression.

6. Inhalation of beclomethasone may cause oral candidiasis and hoarseness. Patients should be advised to rinse the mouth with water after use.

7. Sodium cromoglycate may exacerbate acute asthma and should only be given prophylactically.

Cost

Salbutamol	2 mg	100 tabs =	90p
	4 mg	100 tabs =	£1.70
	2 mg/5 ml syrup	500 ml =	£2.36
	100 microgram inhaler	200 dose =	£2.08
	200 microgram cartridge	100 caps =	£5.30
	400 microgram cartridge	100 caps =	£7.15
Terbutaline	5 mg	100 tabs =	£3.55
	1.5 mg/5 ml syrup	500 ml =	£4.03
	250 microgram inhaler	400 dose =	£5.31
Theophylline s.r.	175 mg (Nuelin)	100 tabs =	£5.22
	250 mg (Nuelin)	100 tabs =	£7.32

Bronchitis

Beclomethasone	50 microgram inhaler	200 dose = £5.56
	100 microgram inhaler	200 dose = £10.56
	250 microgram inhaler	200 dose = £23.10
	100 microgram cartridge	100 caps = £7.56
	200 microgram cartridge	100 caps = £14.35
	400 microgram cartridge	100 caps = £27.27
Prednisolone	1 mg	100 tabs = 45p
	5 mg	100 tabs = 75p
Sodium cromoglycate	5 mg inhaler	112 dose = £14.52
	20 mg cartridge	112 caps = £11.59

Bronchitis

Treatment

Oxytetracycline	Adult dose:	250–500 mg four times daily.
Ampicillin	Adult dose:	250–500 mg four times daily.
	Child dose:	125–250 mg four times daily.
Trimethoprim	Adult dose:	200 mg twice daily.
	Child dose:	6 weeks to 5 months: 25 mg;
		6 months to 5 years: 50 mg;
		6–12 years: 100 mg.
		All twice daily.
Co-trimoxazole	Adult dose:	960 mg twice daily.
	Child dose:	6 weeks to 5 months: 120 mg;

		6 months to 5 years: 240 mg; 6-12 years: 480 mg. All twice daily.
Erythromycin	Adult dose:	250-500 mg four times daily.
	Child dose:	125-250 mg four times daily.
Doxycycline	Adult dose:	200 mg on first day, then 100 mg daily.

Important notes

1. Patients should be urged to stop smoking. Although acute bronchitis may be viral, patients with acute exacerbation of chronic bronchitis do require antibiotics.
2. Tetracyclines should not be used in children under 12 years of age, and should not be used in pregnancy or lactation.
3. Oxytetracycline causes a rise in blood urea in renal impairment, but doxycycline does not. All tetracyclines including doxycycline can cause nausea, vomiting, and diarrhoea.
4. Ampicillin side-effects include urticaria, fever, joint pains, angioneurotic oedema, anaphylactic shock in hypersensitive patients, and diarrhoea. Ampicillin and amoxycillin commonly produce a rash in patients with glandular fever and should not be prescribed if this is suspected. Amoxycillin may be preferred as it causes less diarrhoea and has a three times daily dosage.
5. Neither trimethoprim nor co-trimoxazole should be used in pregnancy or lactation.
6. Co-trimoxazole which is a combination of 5 parts sulphamethoxazole and 1 part trimethoprim may be more effective than trimethoprim alone in haemophilus infections. It may cause nausea, vomiting, rashes, Stevens-Johnson syndrome, agranulocytosis, purpura, and megaloblastic anaemia, particularly in the elderly.
7. Erythromycin may cause nausea, vomiting, abdominal pains, and diarrhoea in high doses.
8. The antibiotics included here are possible alternatives for the treatment of bronchitis, depending on the patient and likely causative bacteria.

Cost

Oxytetracycline	250 mg	100 tabs =	£1.20
Ampicillin	250 mg	100 caps =	£3.35
	500 mg	100 caps =	£7.00
	125 mg/5 ml suspension	500 ml =	£3.80
	250 mg/5 ml suspension	500 ml =	£6.15
Trimethoprim	100 mg	100 tabs =	£3.05
	200 mg	100 tabs =	£4.50
	50 mg/5 ml suspension	500 ml =	£6.90
Co-trimoxazole	480 mg	100 tabs =	£4.85
	240 mg/5 ml suspension	500 ml =	£9.80
Erythromycin	250 mg	100 tabs =	£4.30
	500 mg	100 tabs =	£9.95
	125 mg/5 ml suspension	500 ml =	£7.35
	250 mg/5 ml suspension	500 ml =	£10.85
	500 mg/5 ml suspension	500 ml =	£19.25
Doxycycline	100 mg	100 tabs =	£40.00

Cardiac failure

Treatment

Diuretics
Bendrofluazide   Adult dose: 2.5–10 mg in the morning.

Cardiac failure

Dyazide	Adult dose:	1-4 tabs in the morning.
Frusemide	Adult dose:	20-80 mg in the morning.
Amiloride or	Adult dose:	5-10 mg in the morning.
Spironolactone	Adult dose:	25-100 mg in the morning.

Cardiac glycoside
Digoxin	Adult dose:	62.5-500 micrograms daily.

Potassium replacement
Potassium chloride s.r.	Adult dose:	600-1200 mg three times daily.

Important notes

1. Dyazide is a combination of triamterene 50 mg and hydrochlorthiazide 25 mg.

2. With dyazide, bendrofluazide, and frusemide the serum potassium should be checked at intervals. Potassium supplements may be necessary.

3. Amiloride or spironolactone can be given with frusemide to minimize potassium loss.

4. Bendrofluazide may cause rashes, thrombocytopenia, and impotence.

5. Frusemide may cause rashes.

6. Amiloride may cause rashes and mental confusion.

7. Spironolactone may cause gastro-intestinal disturbances, and gynaecomastia.

8. Digoxin is mainly used for atrial fibrillation. Toxicity is more likely in the elderly, in those with poor renal function, and in hypokalaemia. Check serum digoxin especially if concomitant diuretic therapy. Digoxin may cause anorexia, nausea, vomiting, visual disturbances, arrhythmias, heart block, malaise, and depression.

Cost

Bendrofluazide	2.5 mg	100 tabs =	60p
	5 mg	100 tabs =	25p
Frusemide	20 mg	100 tabs =	80p
	40 mg	100 tabs =	40p
	500 mg	100 tabs =	£30.00
Amiloride	5 mg	100 tabs	£6.80
Spironolactone	25 mg	100 tabs =	£2.70
	50 mg	100 tabs =	£12.00
	100 mg	100 tabs =	£11.00
Dyazide		100 tabs =	£6.50
Digoxin	62.5 micrograms	100 tabs =	40p
	125 micrograms	100 tabs =	30p
	250 micrograms	100 tabs =	45p
Potassium chloride s.r.	600 mg	100 tabs =	50p

Constipation

Treatment

Bulk laxative

Ispaghula husk OTC   Adult dose: 2 teaspoonfuls or 1 sachet in water once or twice daily.
Child dose: $\frac{1}{2}$–1 teaspoonful in water once or twice daily.

Stimulant laxatives

Senna tablets OTC   Adult dose: 7.5–30 mg at night.
Child dose: Half adult dose.

Bisacodyl tablets OTC   Adult dose: 10–20 mg in the morning.
Child dose: 5 mg at night.

Constipation

Faecal softener
Docusate sodium OTC Adult dose: 50–500 mg daily, in divided doses.
Child dose: 12.5–25 mg three times daily.

Osmotic laxative
Lactulose OTC Adult dose: 15 ml twice daily.
Child dose: Under 1 year: 2.5 ml twice daily;
1–5 years: 5 ml twice daily;
6–12 years: 10 ml twice daily.

Suppositories
Glycerol OTC Adult dose: 1 large or medium suppository daily.
Child dose: 1 small suppository daily.

Bisacodyl OTC Adult dose: 10 mg suppos in the morning.
Child dose: 5 mg suppos in the morning.

Important notes

1. Constipation or a change of bowel habit may be the presenting symptom of carcinoma of the bowel.

2. Anal fissure can cause acute constipation in children. Chronic constipation in children often warrants specialist referral.

3. Dietary change to high fibre or regular bran may be the long-term solution. Regular bowel habits are important.

4. All laxatives are contra-indicated if intestinal obstruction is suspected.

5. Ispaghula husk is contra-indicated in faecal impaction and colonic atony: it may cause flatulence and intestinal obstruction.

6. Stimulant laxatives should not be prescribed for prolonged use. They should be avoided in children and pregnancy.

Contraception

7. Docusate may colour urine red, and may cause excoriation and irritation if in prolonged contact with the skin.
8. Glycerol and bisacodyl suppositories are stimulant.

Cost

Ispaghula husk	3.5 g (sachets)	100	=	£7.07
	200 g (granules)	200 g	=	96p
Bisacodyl	5 mg	100 tabs	=	£1.30
	5 mg suppos	12	=	96p
	10 mg suppos	12	=	£1.10
Senna tablets B.P.	7.5 mg	100 tabs	=	50p
Docusate sodium	100 mg	100 tabs	=	£2.55
	50 mg/5 ml syrup	500 ml	=	£3.75
Lactulose	syrup	500 ml	=	£3.85
Glycerol suppositories	small	12	=	42p
	medium	12	=	47p
	large	12	=	55p

Contraception

The Pill

Treatment

Combined

Brevinor/Ovysmen	Dose:	1 daily for 21 days in every 28.
Microgynon 30/ Ovranette	Dose:	1 daily for 21 days in every 28.
Marvelon	Dose:	1 daily for 21 days in every 28.

Phased

Logynon/Trinordiol	Dose:	1 daily for 21 days in every 28.

Progesterone only
Micronor Dose: 1 daily continuously.
Neogest Dose: 1 daily continuously.

Morning-after Pill
Ovran Dose: Two tablets within 72 hours of intercourse, repeated after 12 hours.

Important notes

1. Check blood pressure twice yearly, cervical smear three-yearly.

2. The risk of thrombo-embolic and cardiovascular complications with the combined pill increases with oestrogen content, age, duration of therapy, obesity, smoking, and pre-existing medical conditions. There is also some evidence that the risk of breast cancer may increase with oestrogen content and duration of use.

3. Side-effects of the combined pill are nausea, vomiting, headache, breast tenderness, changes in body weight, thrombosis, changes in libido, depression, chloasma, hypertension, impairment of liver function, benign hepatic tumours, reduced menstrual loss, spotting, and amenorrhoea.

4. Concomitant treatment with broad spectrum antibiotics, carbamazepine, chlordiazepoxide, neomycin, phenobarbitone, phenytoin, primidone, and rifampicin may produce contraceptive failure.

5. Combined preparations are contra-indicated if pregnancy is possible, or with history of thrombo-embolic disease, liver disease, severe migraine, undiagnosed vaginal bleeding, and mammary or endometrial carcinoma.

6. Progesterone-only preparations are to be used with caution in diabetes, hypertension, cardiac disease, functional ovarian cysts, malabsorption syndromes, and severe migraine. They should not be used in pregnancy, liver disease, carcinoma of breast or other sex-hormone-dependent cancers.

7. Other contra-indications include herpes gestationis, deteriorating otosclerosis, and prior to some surgical operations.

8. An expensive alternative to Ovran is Schering PC 4 (4=£1.40).

Cost

Brevinor	3 pack	= £1.56
Logynon	3 pack	= £2.64
Marvelon	3 pack	= £3.90
Microgynon 30	3 pack	= £1.62
Micronor	84 days	= £1.89
Neogest	105 days	= £2.34
Ovran	1 pack	= 37p
Ovranette	3 pack	= £1.86
Ovysmen	3 pack	= £1.59
Trinordiol	3 pack	= £3.28

Depression

Treatment

Tricyclic drugs

Amitriptyline	Adult dose:	50-100 mg at night.
Dothiepin	Adult dose:	75-150 mg at night.
Imipramine	Adult dose:	25-50 mg three times daily.
Clomipramine	Adult dose:	10-150 mg three times daily.

Tetracyclic drug

Mianserin	Adult dose:	10-30 mg three times daily, or as a single dose at night.

Important notes

1. Unhappiness is not a disease.
2. Amitriptyline and dothiepin are sedative. Imipramine is less so.

3. Clomipramine is used for obsessive/compulsive neurosis associated with depression.

4. Tricyclics can cause dry mouth, metallic taste, constipation, nausea, vomiting, weight change, tachycardia, arrhythmias, hypertension, impotence, blurred vision, glaucoma, drowsiness, tremor, fits, extrapyramidal effects, delirium, hypomania, urinary retention, rashes, and blood dyscrasias.

5. Tricyclics interact with a number of drugs including anticholinergics, levodopa, methyldopa, MAOIs.

6. Mianserin has fewer drug interactions; is much less cardiotoxic than the tricyclics but may cause skin rashes, arthralgia, convulsions, headache, and leucopenia. Check WBC after 6 weeks use. It is safer in overdose.

Cost

Amitriptyline	10 mg	100 tabs = £1.10
	25 mg	100 tabs = 40p
	50 mg	100 tabs = £2.40
Dothiepin	25 mg	100 tabs = £4.80
	75 mg	100 tabs = £14.29
Imipramine	10 mg	100 tabs = 70p
	25 mg	100 tabs = 65p
Clomipramine	10 mg	100 tabs = £3.30
	25 mg	100 tabs = £6.45
	50 mg	100 tabs = £12.30
Mianserin	10 mg	100 tabs = £6.55
	20 mg	100 tabs = £13.05
	30 mg	100 tabs = £19.60

Diarrhoea and inflammatory bowel disease

Treatment

Rehydration

Sodium chloride and glucose oral powder OTC   Adult and child dose: 1 powder to 200 ml water, taken liberally.

Antidiarrhoeal

Codeine phosphate   Adult dose: 15–60 mg every 4 to 6 hours.

Loperamide   Adult dose: 4 mg initially, followed by 2 mg after each loose stool for up to 5 days. Maximum 16 mg daily.

Campylobacter enteritis

Erythromycin   Adult dose: 250–500 mg four times daily.

   Child dose: 125–250 mg four times daily.

Inflammatory bowel disease

Sulphasalazine   Adult dose: 500 mg–1 g four times daily.

   Child dose: 20–30 mg/kg daily in divided doses.

Prednisolone   Adult dose: 20 mg in 100 ml retention enema at bedtime for 2 to 4 weeks.

Important notes

1. The basic treatment for acute diarrhoea is rehydration. No solid food or milk for at least 24 hours.

2. Although listed in the *British National Formulary*, the generic form of sodium chloride and glucose powders is rarely available. The chemist may dispense more expensive proprietary preparations.

3. Codeine phosphate is inexpensive and well tried, but may cause drowsiness and exacerbate diverticular disease. Loperamide may cause dizziness or rashes. It should not be used to treat diarrhoea in children.

4. Erythromycin is only used in proven cases of campylobacter enteritis. As a rule antibiotics should not be used in cases of diarrhoea. For erythromycin side-effects, *see under* Bronchitis.

5. Sulphasalazine is only used in proven cases of ulcerative colitis and colonic Crohn's disease. It is a sulphonamide-salicylate combination—beware possible allergy.

6. Prednisolone retention enemas should only be used to treat relapse of inflammatory bowel disease where the diagnosis is established. Be aware of steroid side-effects.

Cost

Sodium chloride and glucose oral powder (Dioralyte)		24 sachets =	£2.40
Codeine phosphate	15 mg	100 tabs =	£1.90
	30 mg	100 tabs =	£1.95
	60 mg	100 tabs =	£6.05
Loperamide	2 mg	100 tabs =	£11.06
Erythromycin	250 mg	100 tabs =	£4.30
	125/5 ml syrup	500 ml =	£6.80
Sulphasalazine	500 mg	100 tabs =	£6.37
Prednisolone retention enema	20 mg/100 ml	7 enemas =	£5.24

Dyspepsia, oesophagitis and peptic ulcer

Treatment

Antacids

Magnesium trisilicate OTC	Adult dose:	5–10 ml or 1 tablet four times daily.
Maalox OTC	Adult dose:	10–20 ml after meals and at bedtime.
	Child dose:	Not used in children.
Aluminium hydroxide OTC	Adult dose:	5–10 ml four times daily.
	Child dose:	Not used in children.
Asilone OTC	Adult dose:	5–10 ml four times daily.
Asilone paediatric suspension OTC	Child dose:	Up to 3 months: 2.5 ml, over 3 months: 5 ml, three to four times daily.
Gaviscon OTC	Adult dose:	10–20 ml four times daily.
	Child dose:	5–10 ml four times daily.
	Infant dose:	$\frac{1}{2}$–1 sachet mixed with feeds.

H_2-receptor blocking drugs

Cimetidine	Adult dose:	400 mg twice daily or 800 mg at night for 4–6 weeks, then 400 mg at night.
	Child dose:	20–40 mg/kg twice daily.
Ranitidine	Adult dose:	150 mg twice daily or 300 mg at night for 4 to 8 weeks, then 150 mg at night.

Dyspepsia, oesophagitis and peptic ulcer

	Child dose:	8 to 18 years: 150 mg twice daily.
Motility modifier **Metoclopramide**	Adult dose: Child dose:	10 mg three times daily. Should not be used in children.

Important notes

1. Recommend small frequent meals, stopping smoking, reduction of alcohol, and improved posture.

2. Four per cent gastric ulcers are malignant. Consider endoscopy, as malignant ulcers may cease producing symptoms initially with H_2-receptor blocking drugs.

3. Aluminium compounds constipate while magnesium compounds are laxative. Maalox is a combination of both. There is concern that long term use of aluminium compounds may be associated with Alzheimer's disease.

4. There is little to choose between the various antacids and they may interfere with other drugs taken concurrently.

5. Cimetidine should be used with caution in renal disease, pregnancy, and with anticoagulants and phenytoin. It may cause gynaecomastia, loss of libido and less commonly rashes, blood dyscrasias, and CNS symptoms.

6. Cimetidine being an enzyme inhibitor may cause reactions when used with other drugs, e.g. diazepam, warfarin, and metoprolol.

7. Ranitidine does not have anti-androgenic effects nor inhibit the metabolism of drugs. It can cause confusion, headaches, constipation, and nausea.

8. Metoclopramide caution: extrapyramidal effects occur particularly in the young, especially females. It enhances the effect of levodopa.

Cost

Magnesium trisilicate	mixture	500 ml	= 55p
	compound tablets	100 tabs	= £1.00
Maalox	suspension	500 ml	= £1.90

Aluminium hydroxide	mixture	500 ml	=	90p
	tablets	100 tabs	=	£1.45
Asilone	500 mg	100 tabs	=	£3.85
	gel	500 ml	=	£1.90
	Suspension	500 ml	=	£1.90
	paediatric suspension	500 ml	=	£5.00
Gaviscon	liquid	500 ml	=	£2.90
	sachets	10 sachets	=	£1.64
	tablets	100 tabs	=	£3.75
Cimetidine	200 mg	100 tabs	=	£14.83
	400 mg	100 tabs	=	£35.52
	800 mg	100 tabs	=	£59.20
Ranitidine	150 mg	100 tabs	=	£49.60
	300 mg	100 tabs	=	£91.43
Metoclopramide	10 mg	100 tabs	=	£2.25

Endocrine conditions

Diabetes mellitus (non-insulin-dependent)

Treatment

Tolbutamide or	Adult dose:	0.5–1.5 g in divided doses.
Glibenclamide	Adult dose:	2.5–15 mg daily in the morning.
Metformin	Adult dose:	500–1000 mg three times daily.

Important notes

1. Diet is the first line of treatment, as obesity is associated with relative insulin resistance.

Endocrine conditions

2. Glibenclamide and tolbutamide may encourage weight gain, should not be used in breast feeding, and should be used with caution in the elderly or in renal failure because of the danger of hypoglycaemia. In the latter two cases tolbutamide is preferred. Sensitivity reactions may occur.

3. Tolbutamide is less likely to cause hypoglycaemia, particularly in the elderly.

4. Use metformin in obese patients but beware of possible lactic acidosis.

Cost

Tolbutamide	500 mg	100 tabs = £1.45
Glibenclamide	2.5 mg	100 tabs = £3.30
	5 mg	100 tabs = £3.70
Metformin	500 mg	100 tabs = £2.38
	850 mg	100 tabs = £3.75

Hypothyroidism

Treatment

Thyroxine   Adult and child dose: 50–200 micrograms daily.

Important notes

1. Caution cardiac conditions.
2. Monitor TSH levels to achieve correct dose, and then review the patient annually.

Cost

Thyroxine	25 micrograms	100 tabs = 35p
	50 micrograms	100 tabs = 20p
	100 micrograms	100 tabs = 25p

Eye conditions

Blepharitis/Conjunctivitis

Treatment

Chloramphenicol eye-drops or ointment — Adults and children: Use every 3-6 hours.

Dry eyes

Treatment

Hypromellose eye-drops OTC — Adults and children: 2 drops every 6 hours.

Dendritic corneal ulcer

Treatment

Idoxuridine eye-drops — Adults and children: 2 drops every 1-4 hours.

Important notes

1. Caution: *Painful red eye* — consider referral.
2. Seek history of foreign body or trauma. Use 1 per cent fluorescein drops to detect corneal abrasion or ulcer. Doctors may wish to refer dendritic ulcers to an ophthalmologist.
3. The hazards of corticosteroid drops are such, that they should never be initiated in general practice.
4. Allergic conditions or dry eyes can cause irritation.
5. Eye-drops are subject to bacterial contamination. Discard them after four weeks.

Cost

Chloramphenicol	eye-drops	10 ml =	67p
	ointment	4 g =	68p
Hypromellose	eye-drops	10 ml =	74p
Idoxuridine	eye-drops	15 ml =	£3.35

Hypertension

Treatment

Diuretic
Bendrofluazide — Adult dose: 2.5–5 mg every morning.
or
Dyazide — Adult dose: 1–2 tabs every morning.

Beta-blockers
Atenolol — Adult dose: 50–100 mg daily.
or
Metroprolol — Adult dose: 50–100 mg twice daily.
or
Propranolol — Adult dose: 10–160 mg twice daily.

Calcium antagonist
Nifedipine s.r. — Adult dose: 20–40 mg twice daily.

ACE inhibitors
Captopril — Adult dose: Initially: 12.5 mg twice daily, usual maintenance dose: 25 mg twice daily.
or
Enalapril — Adult dose: Initially: 5 mg daily, maintenance dose: 10–20 mg daily.

Alpha-blocker
Prazosin   Adult dose: 500 micrograms–20 mg daily, in divided doses.

Centrally-acting
Methyldopa   Adult dose: 250 mg to 1 g four times daily.

Important notes

1. Basic investigations: urea, creatinine, and urinalysis. CXR, ECG, and MSU may be considered appropriate.

2. Underlying conditions such as renal disease, coarctation, Conn's syndrome, etc., warrant referral.

3. Drugs acting in different ways may be used either singly or in combination. Many doctors might commence treatment with bendrofluazide or a beta-blocker and then use them in combination if the blood pressure is not satisfactorily controlled. To this combination nifedipine or ACE inhibitors may be added if necessary. Prazosin or methyldopa may be used for patients in whom the other drugs are contra-indicated or ineffective.

4. Bendrofluazide may cause hypokalaemia, and potassium supplements may be necessary. It may also cause hyperuricaemia, hyperglycaemia, impotence, and skin rash. Dyazide, which is a combination of triamterene 50 mg and hydrochlorthiazide 25 mg, may be preferable in the elderly.

5. Beta-blockers, particularly propranolol, may cause bronchospasm and should not be used in patients with asthma. They may also cause fatigue, bradycardia, vivid dreams, congestive heart failure, Raynaud's phenomenon, impotence, and worsening claudication.

6. Nifedipine may cause throbbing headache, flushing, postural hypotension and tachycardia, and is probably best used in combination with a beta-blocker.

7. ACE inhibitors may cause renal failure in renal artery stenosis (of even mild degree), or angioneurotic oedema. Diuretics must be stopped before treatment. Urea and electrolytes must be checked before and two weeks after commencing treatment.

8. The first dose of prazosin should be small, as it may cause profound hypotension and syncope. Increasing doses should also be small.

9. Methyldopa may cause dry mouth, sedation, depression, drowsiness, diarrhoea, impotence, liver damage, and lupus syndrome. It is contra-indicated in patients with depression, active liver disease, and phaeochromocytoma.

Cost

Bendrofluazide	2.5 mg	100 tabs = 65p
	5 mg	100 tabs = 25p
Dyazide		100 tabs = £6.50
Atenolol	50 mg	100 tabs = £16.96
	100 mg	100 tabs = £23.96
Metroprolol	50 mg	100 tabs = £4.70
	100 mg	100 tabs = £8.75
Propranolol	10 mg	100 tabs = 25p
	40 mg	100 tabs = 40p
	80 mg	100 tabs = 75p
	160 mg s.r.	100 tabs = £1.30
Nifedipine s.r.	20 mg	100 tabs = £19.30
Captopril	12.5 mg	100 tabs = £16.40
	25 mg	100 tabs = £23.88
	50 mg	100 tabs = £36.61
Enalapril	2.5 mg	100 tabs = £20.00
	5 mg	100 tabs = £28.96
	20 mg	100 tabs = £46.80
Prazosin	500 micrograms	100 tabs = £4.30
	1 mg	100 tabs = £5.55
	2 mg	100 tabs = £7.51
Methyldopa	125 mg	100 tabs = £2.25
	250 mg	100 tabs = £3.40
	500 mg	100 tabs = £6.90

Insomnia

Treatment

Temazepam	Adult dose:	10–40 mg at night.
	Elderly patients:	5–15 mg at night.
Nitrazepam	Adult dose:	5–10 mg at night.
	Elderly patients:	2.5–5 mg at night.
Chlormethiazole	Adult dose:	192–500 mg at night.
Promethazine hydrochloride OTC	Adult dose:	25–75 mg at night.
	Child dose:	6–12 months: 10 mg at night;
		1–5 years: 15–20 mg at night;
		6–10 years: 20–25 mg at night.

Important notes

1. The cause of insomnia should be established and underlying factors such as pain, anxiety, or depression should be treated.

2. Hypnotics can cause confusion (especially in the elderly), dependence, hangover, and rebound sleeplessness on withdrawal. They should only be prescribed in short courses for patients with acute distress.

3. Temazepam has a shorter half-life than nitrazepam and therefore causes less hangover. Both can cause drowsiness, dizziness, ataxia, and confusion.

4. Chlormethiazole is less cumulative than nitrazepam and may be safer in elderly patients.

5. Promethazine is an antihistamine and is the only hypnotic suitable for children. Short-term use only is advisable, except in cases of severe pruritus or allergy. Side-effects include drowsiness, irritability, headache, vomiting, and anticholinergic effects such as dry mouth and blurred vision. Paradoxical stimulation may rarely occur.

6. Trimeprazine is no longer recommended as a hypnotic for children.

Cost

Temazepam	10 mg	100 tabs = £1.95
	20 mg	100 tabs = £3.45
	10 mg	100 caps = £2.40
	20 mg	100 caps = £4.15
	10 mg/5 ml elixir	500 ml = £11.40
Nitrazepam	5 mg	100 tabs = 35p
	2.5 mg/5 ml mixture	500 ml = £11.20
Chlormethiazole	192 mg	100 caps = £7.42
	250 mg/5 ml syrup	500 ml = £6.20
Promethazine hydrochloride	10 mg	100 tabs = £1.71
	25 mg	100 tabs = £2.55
	5 mg/5 ml elixir	500 ml = £5.00

Irritable bowel syndrome

Treatment

Mebeverine   Adult dose: 135 mg three times daily before meals.

Important notes

1. Any psychological problems should be discussed with the patient.
2. A high-fibre diet with plentiful fluid intake is advisable.
3. The need for rectal examination, full blood count, liver function tests, faecal occult bloods, barium studies, and endoscopy should be considered before making the diagnosis.
4. Mebeverine is well tolerated and is without serious side-effect.

Cost

Mebeverine   135 mg   100 tabs = £8.35

34   Irritable bowel syndrome

Anal discomfort
Treatment

Anusol OTC   Adult dose: 1 suppository or
or   application of cream
Anusol-HC   twice daily and
                                 after defaecation.

Lignocaine gel   Adult dose: 1 application twice
                                     daily.

Important notes

1. Anal discomfort or pain is a common symptom of patients suffering from haemorrhoids, fissure-in-ano, and proctitis. Patients should be advised to avoid constipation and pay careful attention to local hygiene.
2. Anusol is a mixture of bismuth oxide, bismuth subgallate, zinc oxide, and Peru balsam. Anusol-HC is similar with the addition of hydrocortisone acetate.
3. Lignocaine gel should only be used for short periods as it may cause sensitivity.

Cost

Anusol	cream	23 g	= £1.04
	ointment	25 g	= £1.00
	suppos	12	= £1.06
Anusol-HC	ointment	25 g	= £5.16
	suppos	12	= £2.64
Lignocaine	2 per cent gel	20 g	= 78p
		11 ml	= 95p

Menopause

Treatment

Premarin	Dose:	625 micrograms–2.5 mg daily from 5th to 25th day of cycle.
or **Cycloprogynova** 1 mg or 2 mg	Dose:	One tablet daily from 5th to 26th day of cycle.
Clonidine	Dose:	50 micrograms twice daily.
Dienoestrol cream 0.01%	Dose:	Insert 1–2 applicatorfuls daily for 1–2 weeks, and then 1 applicatorful one to three times weekly as required.

Important notes

1. Most menopausal women do not require hormone replacement therapy or other treatment. Flushing and pruritus vulvae are the two symptoms most amenable to treatment.

2. Premarin consists of conjugated oestrogens whereas cycloprogynova (1 mg) contains oestrogen and progestogen (eleven tablets of oestradiol 1 mg and ten tablets of combined oestradiol 1 mg and levonorgestrel 250 micrograms). Cycloprogynova 2 mg contains double quantity of both drugs.

3. Oestrogen therapy is associated with an increased risk of thromboembolic disease and endometrial carcinoma and possibly breast carcinoma. Progestogens are probably protective against these risks, but are responsible for most of the common side-effects.

4. Women who have had a hysterectomy can be given oestrogens only, whereas others should receive the combined preparation. The combined preparation usually produces withdrawal bleeding, which many women find undesirable. In the absence of withdrawal bleeding

some form of endometrial sampling should be undertaken every two years.

5. In the event of early menopause or hysterectomy, or family history of osteoporotic bone disease, it is desirable that hormone replacement therapy should be given.

6. Prescribing hormone replacement therapy for menopausal women demands the same care as the prescription of the combined contraceptive for younger women. The side-effects and contra-indications are the same (see Contraception).

7. Clonidine may be useful to alleviate flushing in patients unable to take hormone replacement therapy. It can cause dry mouth and sleeplessness and may aggravate depression.

8. Dienoestrol cream is useful local treatment for vaginal dryness or discomfort.

Cost

Premarin	625 micrograms	100 tabs = £4.50
	1.25 mg	100 tabs = £7.30
	2.5 mg	100 tabs = £9.50
Cycloprogynova	1 mg or 2 mg	21 tabs = £3.11
Clonidine	25 micrograms	100 tabs = £5.48
Dienoestrol	0.01% cream	78 g = £2.44

Migraine

Treatment

Metoclopramide	Adult dose:	Under 20 years: 5 mg three times daily. Over 20 years 10 mg three times daily.
	Child dose:	Not recommended for children under 15.

Migraine

Soluble aspirin OTC	Adult dose:	600 mg immediately and six-hourly as required.
or	Child dose:	Not recommended for children under 12.
Soluble paracetamol OTC	Adult dose:	1 g immediately and six-hourly as required.
	Child dose:	6–12 years: 250–500 mg immediately, and six-hourly as required.

Prophylaxis

Clonidine	Adult dose:	50 micrograms twice daily.
Propranolol	Adult dose:	40 mg twice daily.
Pizotifen	Adult dose:	1.5 mg at night or 500 micrograms three times daily.
	Child dose:	Up to 1.5 mg daily; maximum single dose at night 1 mg.

Important notes

1. Elucidate and avoid any precipitating factors. Combined oral contraceptives may cause or worsen migraine.

2. Gastric motility is reduced once the migraine becomes established. Patients should be advised to take metoclopramide, which promotes gastric emptying, immediately at the onset of an attack, and then aspirin or paracetamol 15 minutes later. There is no place for combined preparations of metoclopramide and paracetamol or aspirin.

3. Ergotamine is not favoured in emergency, and metoclopramide injection is preferred.

4. Metoclopramide caution: extrapyramidal effects especially in young people, particularly females.

5. Clonidine, propranolol, and pizotifen are alternative prophylactic drugs.

6. Clonidine can cause dry mouth and sleeplessness and may aggravate depression.

7. Propranolol can cause bronchospasm, peripheral vasoconstriction, and heart failure.

8. Pizotifen can cause weight gain and anti-cholinergic side-effects.

9. Acupuncture may be helpful.

Cost

Soluble aspirin	300 mg	100 tabs =	45p
Soluble paracetamol	500 mg	100 tabs =	£2.16
	120 mg/5 ml suspension	500 ml =	£2.35
	250 mg/5 ml suspension	500 ml =	£5.35
Metoclopramide	10 mg	100 tabs =	£2.25
	5 mg/5 ml syrup	500 ml =	£5.25
	10 mg/2 ml injection	10 amps =	£2.40
Clonidine	25 micrograms	100 tabs =	£5.48
Propranolol	40 mg	100 tabs =	40p
Pizotifen	500 micrograms	100 tabs =	£8.00
	1.5 mg	100 tabs =	£28.50

Mouth infections

Mouth ulcers

Treatment

Hydrocortisone lozenges　　Adult and child dose:　2.5 mg dissolved slowly in the mouth in close contact with the ulcer, four times daily.

Oral candidiasis

Treatment

Nystatin mixture	Child dose:	Instil 1 ml (100 000 units/ml) in the mouth after food, four times daily.
Amphotericin	Adult dose:	Dissolve 10 mg lozenge slowly in mouth four times daily.

Important notes

1. Nystatin mixture should not be washed away with drinks.
2. Treatment should continue for 2 days after the infection is cleared.

Herpetic stomatitis/Herpes labialis

Treatment

Idoxuridine 0.1% drops	Adults and older children:	Hold 2 ml in contact with lesions for 3 minutes four times daily.
	Younger children:	Paint lesions four times daily.
Acyclovir cream	Adult and child dose:	Apply to lesions every four hours for 5 days.

Important notes

1. Oral and perioral herpes do not usually require specific treatment.
2. There is concern that the use of acyclovir for the treatment of such minor conditions may lead to the development of drug-resistant viruses.
3. Idoxuridine 0.1 per cent drops are the eye-drops and not the skin paint.
4. Acyclovir cream should be applied to lesions on the lips sparingly.

40 Mouth infections

Oral hygiene

Treatment

Chlorhexidine 0.2% OTC	Adult and child dose:	Rinse mouth with 10 ml for 1 minute twice daily.

Dental abscess

Treatment

Penicillin V	Adult dose:	250 mg four times daily.
	Child dose:	1–5 years: 125 mg four times daily; 6–12 years: 250 mg four times daily.
Metronidazole	Adult dose:	200 mg three times daily.
	Child dose:	7.5 mg/kg every eight hours, daily.

Important notes

1. Most dental infections seem to respond to simple penicillin. Erythromycin may be used for patients allergic to penicillin.

2. Metronidazole may be given if anaerobic infection is suspected or if the condition fails to respond to penicillin. Dental abscesses are best treated by dentists.

Cost

Hydrocortisone lozenges	2.5 mg	100 tabs	= £7.00
Nystatin mixture	100 000 units/ml	30 ml	= £2.50
Amphotericin lozenges	10 mg	100 tabs	= £6.60
Idoxuridine 0.1% drops		15 ml	= £3.35

Acyclovir	cream	2 g	= £6.33
		10 g	= £19.07
Chlorhexidine 0.2%	mouthwash	500 ml	= £2.08
Penicillin V	125 mg	100 tabs	= £1.10
	250 mg	100 tabs	= £1.65
	125 mg/5 ml elixir	500 ml	= £2.65
Metronidazole	200 mg	100 caps	= £2.90
	200 mg/5 ml suspension	500 ml	= £20.64

Nausea and/or vomiting and/or vertigo

Treatment

Prochlorperazine	Adult dose:	12.5–25 mg immediately in acute vomiting/vertigo, then 5–10 mg orally 2–4 hours later. Maintenance dose: 5 mg three times daily.
	Child dose:	1–5 years: 2.5 mg twice daily; 6–12 years: 5 mg twice to three times daily.

Important notes

1. Check cause of nausea, vomiting, or vertigo.
2. Prochlorperazine may cause dry mouth, and sedation particularly with alcohol, mainly in high dosage. It can also cause extrapyramidal effects especially in young people, particularly females.

3. It can cause hypotension in elderly patients.

4. Initial dosage to adults can be either 12.5 mg by intramuscular injection or 25 mg rectally as a suppository. In severe vomiting a child may be given a 5 mg suppository.

Cost

Prochlorperazine			
	5 mg	100 tabs	= £1.90
	10 mg	100 tabs	= £3.75
	5 mg/5 ml syrup	500 ml	= £8.00
	5 mg suppositories	10 suppos	= £4.00
	25 mg suppositories	10 suppos	= £5.26
	12.5 mg/ml injection	10 × 1 ml	= £3.10

Neurological disorders

Epilepsy

Treatment

Phenytoin   Adult dose: 150–300 mg daily can be increased slowly to 600 mg.

Carbamazepine Adult dose: 100–200 mg once or twice daily, can be increased to 0.8–1.2 g daily.

Important notes

1. General practitioners do not normally initiate the treatment of epilepsy except in known cases of cerebrovascular or neoplastic disease in adults.

2. Both drugs can cause dizziness, drowsiness, and gastro-intestinal disturbance.

Neurological disorders

3. Phenytoin can cause headache, confusion, and insomnia. It can also cause a variety of skin problems, gingival hypertrophy, and anaemia due to folate deficiency.

4. Carbamazepine can cause a generalized erythematous rash in 3 per cent of patients, and leucopenia can rarely occur.

5. Correct dosages can only be achieved by monitoring plasma concentration.

Neuralgia

Treatment

Analgesics	*See under* Pain.
Carbamazepine	*See above*—epilepsy.

Important note

1. Tricyclic antidepressants may be valuable in treating post-herpetic neuralgia.

Spasticity

Treatment

Diazepam	Adult dose:	2–5 mg three times daily.
Baclofen	Adult dose:	5–30 mg three times daily.

Important notes

1. Diazepam is a benzodiazepine. For side-effects, *see under* Anxiety.

2. Baclofen may cause nausea, vomiting, fatigue, and hypotension. It should be used with caution in patients with psychiatric illness and cerebrovascular disease.

Parkinsonism

Treatment

Orphenadrine	Adult dose:	150 mg gradually increased to maximum 400 mg, in three or four divided doses.
Sinemet	Adult dose:	100 mg levodopa three or four times daily, increased to 750 mg to 1.5 g, in divided doses.
Madopar	Adult dose:	50–100 mg twice daily, increased to 400–800 mg, in divided doses.

Important notes

1. Identify causative drugs (e.g. phenothiazines, methyldopa) and eliminate if possible.

2. Orphenadrine should be used with care in patients with prostatic disease, glaucoma, hepatic or renal impairment. Dry mouth may be a problem and cardiovascular disease may be a contra-indication.

3. Orphenadrine is usually prescribed to counteract phenothiazine side-effects.

4. Sinemet is a combination of levodopa and carbidopa, and Madopar is a combination of levodopa and benserazide. Doses are expressed as levodopa.

5. Levodopa appears to have a limited span of therapeutic effect and its use should be kept in reserve and carefully evaluated. Its side-effects include anorexia, nausea, insomnia, cardiac arrhythmias, hypotension, discoloration of body fluids, and abnormal movements as well as psychiatric symptoms.

6. Levodopa preparations should be used with caution in patients suffering from peptic ulcer, cardiovascular disease, diabetes, open angle glaucoma, skin melanoma, and psychiatric illness.

Cost

Phenytoin	25 mg	100 caps = £1.95
	50 mg	100 caps = £2.00
	100 mg	100 caps = £2.15
Carbamazepine	100 mg	100 tabs = £2.65
	200 mg	100 tabs = £4.95
	400 mg	100 tabs = £10.05
Diazepam	2 mg	100 tabs = 10p
Baclofen	10 mg	100 tabs = £11.70
Orphenadrine	50 mg	100 tabs = £1.50
Sinemet	'110' 100 mg levodopa	100 tabs = £8.55
	'Plus' 100 mg levodopa	100 tabs = £12.60
	'275' 250 mg levodopa	100 tabs = £17.87
Madopar	'62.5' 50 mg levodopa	100 caps = £5.94
	'125' 100 mg levodopa	100 caps = £13.50
	'250' 200 mg levodopa	100 caps = £22.45

Otitis externa

Treatment

Locorten-vioform drops	Adult and child dose:	Instil 2-3 drops twice daily.
or Otosporin drops	Adult and child dose:	Instil 2-3 drops three times daily.

Important notes

1. Caution: local effects due to strong steroid preparations. Fungal overgrowth and local sensitivity reactions may occur with prolonged use of anti-infective agents.

2. Locorten-vioform is a mixture of clioquinol 1 per cent and flumethasone pivalate 0.02 per cent.

3. Otosporin is a mixture of hydrocortisone 1 per cent, neomycin sulphate 0.439 per cent and polymyxin B sulphate 0.119 per cent.

Ear wax

Treatment

Olive-oil drops OTC   Adult and child dose: Instil 2 drops four times daily.

Important note

1. In the event of suspected otitis media ear-drops are contra-indicated and a suitable oral antibiotic should be given (*see* Upper respiratory tract infection).

Cost

Locorten-vioform	7.5 ml = £1.05
Otosporin	5 ml = £4.09
	10 ml = £6.99
Olive oil	10 ml = 5p

Pain

Treatment

Soluble aspirin OTC	Adult dose:	300–600 mg four/six-hourly as necessary.
	Child dose:	Contra-indicated for children under 12 years of age.
Paracetamol OTC	Adult dose:	500 mg to 1 g four/six-hourly as necessary.

Pain   47

	Child dose:	Under 3 months: not recommended. 3 months to 1 year: 60–220 mg; 1–6 years: 120–240 mg; 6–12 years: 250–500 mg. All six-hourly as necessary.
Co-codaprin OTC	Adult dose:	1–2, four to six hourly if necessary.
	Child dose	Not suitable for children.
Co-codamol OTC	Adult dose:	1–2, four to six hourly if necessary.
Co-proxamol	Adult dose:	1–2, six hourly as necessary.
Co-dydramol	Adult dose:	1–2, four to six hourly as necessary.
Dihydrocodeine	Adult dose:	30 mg four to six hourly as necessary.
Pethidine	Adult dose:	50–150 mg four hourly as necessary.

Important notes

1. Arranged in escalating order of analgesic potency.
2. Aspirin must not be given to children under 12 years old.
3. Constipation can be caused by all codeine derivatives.
4. Co-codaprin is aspirin 400 mg and codeine phosphate 8 mg.
   Co-codamol is paracetamol 500 mg and codeine phosphate 8 mg.
   Co-proxamol is paracetamol 325 mg and dextropropoxyphene 32.5 mg.
   Co-dydramol is paracetamol 500 mg and dihydrocodeine 10 mg.
5. Pethidine is mainly used in renal colic and childbirth.
6. Dependency is a significant hazard of long-term use of codeine, dihydrocodeine, dextropropoxyphene, and pethidine. Dextropropoxyphene is especially dangerous in overdose particularly with alcohol.

Night Cramps

Treatment

Quinine sulphate   Adult dose: 300 mg at night.

Important note

The dose should not be exceeded and no other pain is helped by quinine sulphate. Side-effects are rare at this dose, but can include abdominal pain, nausea, and headaches.

Cost

Soluble aspirin	300 mg	100 tabs =	45p
Paracetamol	500 mg	100 tabs =	40p
	120 mg/5 ml suspension	500 ml =	£2.35
	250 mg/5 ml suspension	500 ml =	£5.15
Co-codaprin		100 tabs =	£1.20
	dispersible	100 tabs =	£1.55
Co-codamol		100 tabs =	£1.40
	dispersible	100 tabs =	£2.45
Co-proxamol		100 tabs =	£1.40
Co-dydramol		100 tabs =	£1.65
Dihydrocodeine	30 mg	100 tabs =	£3.10
	10 mg/5 ml elixir	500 ml =	£4.27
Pethidine hydrochloride	50 mg	100 tabs =	£1.46
Quinine sulphate	300 mg	100 tabs =	£3.60

Premenstrual syndrome

Treatment

Bendrofluazide	Adult dose:	5 mg daily on days 16-28 of menstrual cycle.
Pyridoxine OTC	Adult dose:	50 mg twice daily on days 16-28 of menstrual cycle.
Norethisterone	Adult dose:	5 mg twice daily on days 19-26 of menstrual cycle.
Dydrogesterone	Adult dose:	10 mg twice daily on days 12-26 of menstrual cycle.

Important notes

1. Salt restriction and/or a diuretic may be useful for bloating.
2. Pyridoxine is useful for depression and irritation.
3. Be aware that premenstrual syndrome can be a symptom of other psychiatric or psychosexual problems.
4. Norethisterone and dydrogesterone should be used with caution in diabetes, hypertension, and hepatic or renal disease, and may cause acne, urticaria, oedema, gastro-intestinal upsets, changes in libido, breast discomfort, and irregular menstruation.
5. Some patients are said to obtain relief with oil of evening primrose. However, this can only be prescribed on the NHS for eczema.

Dysmenorrhoea

Treatment

Mefenamic acid	Adult dose:	250-500 mg three times daily.
Dydrogesterone	Adult dose:	10 mg twice daily on days 5-12 of menstrual cycle.

Important notes

1. Mefenamic acid may be better than simple analgesics.
2. Mefenamic acid can cause gastric irritation, hypersensitivity reactions (including asthma), headache, drowsiness, renal impairment, rashes, and blood dyscrasias.
3. Combined oral contraceptives may also prevent dysmenorrhoea.

Cost

Bendrofluazide	5 mg	100 tabs = 21p
Pyridoxine	10 mg	100 tabs = £1.60
	20 mg	100 tabs = £1.30
	50 mg	100 tabs = £2.60
Norethisterone	5 mg	100 tabs = £9.60
Dydrogesterone	10 mg	100 tabs = £16.75
Mefenamic acid	250 mg	100 caps = £4.70
	500 mg	100 tabs = £10.50

Pruritus vulvae/vaginal discharge

Treatment

Nystatin pessaries	Adult:	1 pessary (100 000 units) to be inserted at night for 14 nights.
and **Nystatin cream**	Adult:	100 000 units/g apply twice daily.
Clotrimazole pessaries	Adult:	100 mg at night for 6 nights, or 200 mg at night for 3 nights.
and **Clotrimazole cream 1%**	Adult:	Apply twice daily.

Pruritis vulvae/vaginal discharge 51

| Metronidazole | Adult: | 400 mg twice daily for 5–7 days. |
| Doxycycline | Adult: | 200 mg as an initial dose and then 100 mg daily for 14 days. |

Important notes

1. Ideally high vaginal and cervical swabs should be taken to exclude/discover trichomonal or other venereal infection. If no response to treatment, swabs are essential.

2. Nystatin and clotrimazole are used for candida, metronidazole for trichomonas and gardnerella, and doxycycline for chlamydia infections.

3. Consider treating partner or suggest he sees his own doctor.

4. Diabetes, pregnancy, steroids, antibiotics, and the pill are predisposing causes of candidiasis, and recurrence is more likely in these conditions.

5. Nystatin and clotrimazole creams may be used in combination with pessaries for associated vulvitis (or partner's balanitis) and may produce local irritation. This may be relieved by combination with hydrocortisone.

6. Metronidazole impairs the metabolism of alcohol, which must be avoided. It should not be used in pregnancy or breast feeding. Side-effects include gastro-intestinal disturbances, headache, vertigo, ataxia, confusion, seizures, peripheral neuropathy, skin rashes, and neutropenia.

7. Doxycycline may cause nausea, vomiting, and diarrhoea.

Cost

Nystatin pessaries with applicator		15 pessaries	= £1.09
Nystatin cream	60 g	1 tube	= £3.26
Clotrimazole pessaries with applicator	100 mg	6 pessaries	= £2.64
	200 mg	3 pessaries	= £2.58
	500 mg	1 pessary	= £2.58
Clotrimazole cream	35 g	1 tube	= £5.22
Metronidazole	200 mg	100 tabs	= £2.90

Skin conditions

Acute eczema/Dermatitis

Treatment

Betamethasone 0.1% cream or ointment	Adult and child dose:	Apply twice daily.

Dry eczema/Ichthyosis

Treatment

Aqueous cream OTC	Adult and child:	Apply twice daily.
Oilatum OTC	Adult and child:	Use liberally in the bath.
Hydrocortisone 1% ointment OTC	Adult and child:	Apply twice daily.
Emulsifying ointment OTC	Adult and child:	Use as soap substitute in the bath.
Dimethicone cream OTC	Adult and child:	Use as barrier cream.

Nappy rash

Treatment

Zinc cream OTC	All ages:	Apply with each nappy change.
Nystaform-HC cream	All ages:	Apply twice daily.

Psoriasis

Treatment

Alphosyl cream OTC	Adult and child:	Apply up to four times daily.

Skin conditions 53

Dithrocream (0.1%, 0.25%)	Adult and child:	Apply for 30 minutes daily in increasing strengths.
Betamethasone 0.025% cream or ointment	Adult and child:	Apply daily.
Polytar liquid OTC	Adult and child:	Shampoo twice weekly.

Important notes

1. Creams are either water-miscible and easily washed off or oily. They tend to moisten the skin although modern ointment bases have occlusive properties on the skin surface and may encourage hydration.

2. Potent steroid preparations damage subcutaneous collagen and should never be used on the face.

3. Nystaform-HC cream is a combination of hydrocortisone 0.05 per cent, nystatin 100 000 u/g, and chlorhexidine 1 per cent.

4. Alphosyl cream is a combination of coal tar extract 5 per cent and allantoin 2 per cent.

5. Dithrocream may produce local burning sensation and stain skin, hair, and clothing. Treatment should be started with the weakest preparation, and the strength increased as tolerated.

6. Exacerbation of eczema may be caused by local bacterial infection. This should be treated with local or systemic antibiotics.

Cost

Alphosyl cream		75 g	= £1.56
Aqueous cream		100 g	= 28p
Betamethasone (0.025% cream or ointment)		100 g	= £4.12
Betamethasone (0.1% cream or ointment)		100 g	= £3.95
Dimethicone cream		100 g	= 54p
Dithrocream	0.1%	100 g	= £6.72
	0.25%	100 g	= £7.24

54   Skin infections

Oilatum	40 g	= £1.79
Emulsifying ointment	100 g	= 30p
Hydrocortisone 1% ointment	100 g	= £1.94
Nystaform-HC cream	30 g	= £2.73
Polytar liquid	350 ml	= £2.37
Zinc cream	100 g	= 36p

Skin infections

Impetigo

Treatment

Chlortetracycline 3% cream	Adult and child:	Apply twice daily.
Flucloxacillin	Adult dose:	250 mg four times daily.
	Child dose:	Up to 2 years: 62.5 mg four times daily; 2-10 years: 125 mg both four times daily.

Important note

Systemic antibiotics are sometimes necessary for impetigo.

Cellulitis

Treatment

Penicillin V	Adult dose:	250-500 mg four times daily.
	Child dose:	Up to 1 year: 62.5 mg; 1-5 years: 125 mg; 6-12 years: 250 mg. All four times daily.

Skin infections 55

Flucloxacillin	Adult dose:	250–500 mg four times daily.
	Child dose:	Up to 1 year: 62.5 mg; 1–5 years: 125 mg; 6–12 years: 250 mg. All four times daily.

Erysipelas

Treatment

Penicillin V	Adult dose:	250–500 mg four times daily.
	Child dose:	Up to 1 year: 62.5 mg; 1–5 years: 125 mg; 6–12 years: 250 mg. All four times daily.

Acne vulgaris

Treatment

Oxytetracycline	Adult dose:	250 mg four times daily for 1–4 weeks, then twice daily as long as condition recurs.
	Child dose:	Inappropriate under 12 years of age.
Co-trimoxazole	Adult dose:	480 mg twice daily for 1–4 weeks, then once daily as long as condition recurs.
	Child dose:	Inappropriate under 12 years of age.
Erythromycin	Adult dose:	250 mg four times daily for 1–4 weeks, then twice daily as long as condition recurs.
Benzoyl peroxide 5% or 10% lotion OTC		Apply daily after cleansing.

Furunculosis

Treatment

Chlorhexidine liquid soap OTC	
Chlorhexidine gluconate 4% in an emulsion base OTC	Use as soap substitute.

Important notes

1. For side-effects of oxytetracycline, co-trimoxazole, and erythromycin, *see under* Bronchitis. Be particularly aware of possibility of pregnancy in young women.

2. Long term use of co-trimoxazole may lead to folic acid deficiency.

3. Organisms resistant to all antibiotics particularly erythromycin may occur with long term use.

4. Benzoyl peroxide may be used alone or in addition to one of the antibiotics suggested.

Scabies

Treatment

Benzyl benzoate 25% application OTC	Adult dose:	Apply two nights running over whole body except neck and head.
Lindane 1% lotion OTC	Child dose:	Apply once over whole body except neck and head. Repeat in five days.

Important notes

1. The irritation of scabies is a hypersensitivity response to the insect's waste products. It can be present without apparent itching. Look for burrows.

2. Benzyl benzoate is itself irritating to skin and children are better treated with lindane.

Tinea

Treatment

Whitfield's ointment OTC	Adult and child dose:	Apply twice daily.
Clotrimazole 1% cream	Adult and child dose:	Apply twice daily.

Herpes simplex

Treatment

Betadine paint (povidone-iodine 10%) OTC	Adult and child dose:	Apply twice daily.
Acyclovir cream	Adult and child dose:	Apply five times daily.

Herpes zoster

Treatment

Idoxuridine 5% application	Adult and child dose:	Apply four times daily for five days.
Acyclovir cream	Adult and child dose:	Apply five times daily.
Acyclovir	Adult and child dose:	800 mg five times daily for seven days.

Warts

Treatment

Salicyclic acid collodion OTC	Adult and child:	Apply daily.

Important notes

1. Acyclovir cream must be used early to be effective.
2. Systemic acyclovir should only be used in general practice for the treatment of ophthalmic shingles, or exceptionally for severely debilitated patients.

Skin infections

3. There is no evidence that acyclovir reduces the incidence or duration of post-herpetic neuralgia.
4. Warts are viral in origin and resolve spontaneously.

Cost

Acyclocir	800 mg	35 tabs	= £113.00
Acyclovir	5% cream	2 g	= £6.33
		10 g	= £19.07
Benzoyl peroxide	5% lotion	150 ml	= £5.15
	10% lotion	150 ml	= £5.45
Benzyl benzoate	25% application	500 ml	= £1.84
Betadine paint		8 ml	= 69p
Chlortetracycline	3% cream	30 g	= £1.82
Clotrimazole	1% cream	20 g	= £1.82
Co-trimoxazole	480 mg	100 tabs	= £4.85
	240 mg/5 ml suspension	500 ml	= £9.80
Erythromycin	250 mg	100 tabs	= £4.30
	500 mg	100 tabs	= £9.95
	250 mg/5 ml suspension	500 ml	= £10.85
	500 mg/5 ml suspension	500 ml	= £19.25
Flucloxacillin	250 mg	100 caps	= £13.50
	500 mg	100 caps	= £28.00
	125 mg/5 ml syrup	500 ml	= £16.45
Idoxuridine	5% application	5 ml	= £4.90
Lindane	1% lotion	500 ml	= £2.08
Oxytetracycline	250 mg	100 tabs	= £1.20
Penicillin V	125 mg	100 tabs	= £1.05
	250 mg	100 tabs	= £1.65
Salicyclic acid collodion		5 ml	= 5p
Whitfield's ointment		100 g	= 60p

Terminal care—symptom control

Much of the advice that appears below applies to the care of patients with malignant disease. In time general practitioners may need to become familiar with the treatment of AIDs.

Pain

1. The aim is to maintain the patient free of pain at all times. The dose of administration, and potency of analgesics should be escalated using mild analgesics initially (*see* section on pain).

2. High doses of opiates may be required, increasing strength of administration as necessary, to *prevent* the recurrence of pain or distress. The median dose of oral morphine is 120 mg per day—very few patients require more than 600 mg per day. A syringe pump delivering subcutaneous morphine/diamorphine enables continuous administration for symptom relief.

3. Bone pain may be relieved by NSAID's (*see* section on arthritis).

4. Oral: parenteral potency ratios: 3 mg oral morphine=2 mg oral diamorphine=1 mg injectable diamorphine or 1.5 mg injectable morphine.

Treatment

Morphine sulphate s.r.	Adult dose:	10 mg upwards twice daily.
Morphine or **diamorphine solution**	Adult dose:	5 mg upwards four hourly.
Morphine or **diamorphine (by injection)**	Adult dose:	10 mg upwards four hourly or total daily requirement by syringe pump over 24 hours.

Nausea and vomiting

1. Many cases respond to simple anti-emetics (*see* section nausea and/or vomiting).

2. The nausea associated with opiates often improves over 7 to 14 days. Very low dose haloperidol (1.5–3 mg at night) is the anti-emetic of choice for opioid-induced vomiting.

3. Domperidone is particularly helpful for the control of nausea/vomiting associated with cytotoxic drug therapy.

4. Cyclizine may be helpful in nausea associated with hepatic secondary involvement. It is also available for parenteral use combined with morphine.

Treatment

Haloperidol	Adult dose:	1.5–3 mg at night.
Domperidone	Adult dose:	10–20 mg eight hourly. Rectally: 30–60 mg eight hourly.
	Child dose:	100 micrograms per kilogram eight hourly. Rectally: 200 mg/per kilogram eight hourly.
Cyclizine	Adult dose:	150 mg eight hourly.
	Child dose:	2–5 years: 12.5 mg eight hourly. 6–12 years: 25 mg eight hourly.

Constipation and diarrhoea

1. Constipation is associated with the administration of opiates, but this should not be a problem if a combination of a stimulant laxative with a faecal softener are used early enough. Bulk laxatives are contraindicated (*see* section on constipation).

2. Faecal impaction should be preventable, but should it occur disposable enemas of sodium citrate may be needed.

3. Patients with pelvic malignancy may suffer from diarrhoea, and loperamide is the drug of choice (*see* section on diarrhoea).

Treatment

Sodium citrate enema	Adult dose:	5 ml compound enema pack.

Anorexia

1. Corticosteroids such as prednisolone or dexamethasone stimulate appetite.

Treatment

Prednisolone	Adult dose:	30 mg daily.
Dexamethasone	Adult dose:	2 mg twice daily.

Restlessness and confusion

1. Chlorpromazine (see under Agitation) controls restlessness and confusion and can also relieve nausea.

Raised intracranial pressure

1. Presents with a variety of symptoms from primary or secondary tumours, most frequently diplopia, headache, and psychological symptoms.

Treatment

Dexamethasone	Adult dose:	2–16 mg daily in divided doses.

Dry mouth/fungal infection

1. Simple mouthwashes and good nursing care can prevent discomfort.
2. Fungal infections are common, particularly candida (see mouth infections).
3. Glycerine mouthwash should never be given undiluted since this dehydrates the oral mucosa.

Treatment

Compound thymol glycerin mouthwash	Adult dose:	Diluted up to three times with water.

Respiratory symptoms

1. Cough and dyspnoea may be relieved by simple remedies (*see* section URTI). Intractable cough and dyspnoea require opiates.
2. Excessive respiratory secretions can be ameliorated by subcutaneous injection of hyoscine hydrobromide.

Treatment

Hyoscine hydrobromide	Adult dose:	200 micrograms six hourly.

Cost

Morphine sulphate s.r.	10 mg	100 tabs	= £12.83
	30 mg	100 tabs	= £30.82
	60 mg	100 tabs	= £60.00
	100 mg	100 tabs	= £95.17
Morphine solution		500 ml	= £8.40
Diamorphine solution		500 ml	= £8.40
Morphine injection	10 mg	1 amp	= 37p
	15 mg	1 amp	= 37p
	30 mg	1 amp	= 37p
Haloperidol	500 micrograms	100 tabs	= £2.20
	1.5 mg	100 tabs	= £4.16
Domperidone	10 mg	100 tabs	= £10.87
	5 mg/5 ml	500 ml	= £4.50
	30 mg suppos	10 suppos	= £2.64
Cyclizine	50 mg	10 tabs	= £3.75
	50 mg/1 ml injection 1 amp		= 43p
Sodium citrate enema	5 ml compound pack	1 pack	= 30p
Prednisolone	5 mg	100 tabs	= 75p
Dexamethasone	2 mg	100 tabs	= £8.65
Compound Thymol	Mouth wash		
Glycerine mouthwash	Solution tabs	20 tabs	= 26p
Hyoscine hydrobromide	300 micrograms	100 tabs	= £1.15
	400 micrograms/ml injection	1 amp	= 81p

Upper respiratory tract infections

The common cold

Treatment

Needs no specific treatment.

Catarrh

Treatment

Steam inhalations		Three-hourly as required.
Pseudoephedrine OTC	Adult dose:	60 mg three times daily.
	Child dose:	Under 2 years not recommended; 2-5 years: 2.5 ml; 6-12 years: 5 ml. All three times daily.

Important notes

1. At least two weeks blocked nose without facial pain or purulent discharge = catarrh.
2. Beware allergies, sinusitis, polyps.
3. Fresh air and lower setting on central heating may be an effective treatment.
4. Hot water (not boiling) for inhalation. Beware spilling, particularly for elderly people and children.
5. Pseudoephedrine should be avoided in patients with hypertension, hyperthyroidism, coronary heart disease, and diabetes. It is totally contra-indicated for patients on MAOI inhibitors, and can cause insomnia if taken in the evening.

Cough

Treatment

Codeine linctus OTC	Adult dose:	5-10 ml up to four times daily.
Codeine linctus paediatric OTC	Child dose:	1-5 years: 5 ml up to four times daily.
Simple linctus OTC	Adult dose:	5-10 ml up to four times daily.
Simple linctus paediatric OTC	Child dose:	5-10 ml up to four times daily.

Important note

Simple linctus is palliative for sore throats but codeine linctus is a cough suppressant and should not be used if a cough is productive. It is not generally recommended for children.

Sinusitis

Treatment

Ampicillin	Adult dose:	250-500 mg four times daily.
	Child dose:	125-250 mg four times daily.
Erythromycin	Adult dose:	250-500 mg six hourly daily.
	Child dose:	Under 2 years: 125 mg; 2-8 years: 250 mg; Over 8 years: 500 mg. All four times daily.
Doxycycline	Adult dose:	200 mg on first day then 100 mg daily.

Important notes

1. Sinusitis must be differentiated from simple catarrh, and is characterized by fever, facial pain, sinus tenderness, and mucopurulent nasal discharge.

2. For patients allergic to penicillins, erythromycin, or doxycycline are suitable alternatives.

3. For side-effects of ampicillin, erythromycin and doxycycline *see under* Bronchitis.

Throat infections

Treatment

Paracetamol OTC	Adult dose:	500 mg four–six-hourly if necessary.
	Child dose:	Under 1 year: 60–120 mg; 1–5 years: 120–250 mg; 6–12 years: 250–500 mg. All four times daily.
Penicillin V	Adult dose:	250–500 mg four times daily.
	Child dose:	Under 1 year: 62.5 mg; 1–5 years: 125 mg; 6–12 years: 250 mg. All four times daily.
Erythromycin	Adult dose:	250–500 mg four times daily.
	Child dose:	Under 2 years: 125 mg; 2–8 years: 250 mg; Over 8 years: 500 mg. All four times daily.

Important notes

1. 70 per cent or more of throat infections are viral and require only symptomatic treatment.

2. Paracetamol is used to treat discomfort and pyrexia in viral or bacterial conditions.

3. Penicillin V is the treatment of choice for bacterial conditions and erythromycin the first alternative if the patient is allergic to penicillin.

4. Side-effects of penicillin and erythromycin are listed in the section on bronchitis.

Otitis media

Treatment

Ampicillin	Adult dose:	500 mg four times daily.
	Child dose:	250 mg four times daily.
Amoxycillin	Adult dose:	250–500 mg three times daily.
	Child dose:	Under 10 years: 125 mg three times daily.
Co-trimoxazole	Adult dose:	960 mg twice daily.
	Child dose:	6 weeks to 6 months: 120 mg twice daily; 6 months to 5 years: 240 mg twice daily; 6–12 years: 480 mg twice daily.
Erythromycin	Adult dose:	250–500 mg four times daily.
	Child dose:	Under 2 years: 125 mg; 2–8 years: 250 mg; Over 8 years: 500 mg. All four times daily.

Important notes

1. Amoxycillin and ampicillin have an identical spectrum of antibacterial activity. Amoxycillin is only indicated in treatment of acute otitis media in children under 4 years of age.

2. Side-effects of amoxycillin and ampicillin are similar although diarrhoea is less common with amoxycillin. For side-effects of other antibiotics *see* in section on bronchitis.

Cost

Steam inhalations		Free	
Pseudoephedrine	60 mg	100 tabs =	£5.85
	30 mg/5 ml syrup	500 ml =	£4.75
Codeine linctus		500 ml =	£1.75

Upper respiratory tract infections

Codeine linctus paediatric		500 ml	=	90p
Simple linctus		500 ml	=	80p
Simple linctus paediatric		500 ml	=	80p
Ampicillin	250 mg	100 caps	=	£3.35
	500 mg	100 caps	=	£7.00
	125 mg/5 ml suspension	500 ml	=	£3.80
	250 mg/5 ml suspension	500 ml	=	£6.15
Paracetamol	500 mg	100 tabs	=	40p
	120 mg/5 ml suspension	500 ml	=	£2.35
Penicillin V	125 mg	100 tabs	=	£1.05
	250 mg	100 tabs	=	£1.65
	62.5 mg/5 ml syrup	500 ml	=	£2.00
	125 mg/5 ml	500 ml	=	£3.65
	250 mg/5 ml	500 ml	=	£4.10
Amoxycillin	250 mg	100 caps	=	£13.85
	500 mg	100 caps	=	£28.00
	125 mg/5 ml syrup	100 ml	=	£8.75
	250 mg/5 ml	100 ml	=	£16.30
Co-trimoxazole	480 mg	100 tabs	=	£4.85
	240 mg/5 ml suspension	500 ml	=	£9.80
Erythromycin	250 mg	100 tabs	=	£4.30
	500 mg	100 tabs	=	£9.95
	125 mg/5 ml suspension	500 ml	=	£7.35
	250 mg/5 ml suspension	500 ml	=	£10.85
	500 mg/5 ml suspension	500 ml	=	£19.25

Urinary tract conditions

Acute infection

Treatment

Trimethoprim
Adult dose: 200 mg twice daily.
Child dose: 2–5 months: 25 mg twice daily;
6 months to 5 years: 50 mg twice daily;
6–12 years: 100 mg twice daily.

Ampicillin
Adult dose: 500 mg four times daily.
Child dose: 250 mg four times daily.

Nitrofurantoin
Adult dose: 100 mg four times daily.
Child dose: 3 months to 2 years: 12.5 mg four times daily;
2–6 years: 25 mg four times daily;
6–11 years: 50 mg four times daily;
11–14 years: 74 mg four times daily.

Nalidixic acid
Adult dose: 1 g every six hours for seven days, reducing to 500 mg every six hours.
Child dose: Not recommended under 3 months.
3 months–12 years: 50 mg/kg body weight daily.

Important notes

1. Ideally, send MSU before and after treatment.

Urinary tract conditions

2. Trimethoprim may cause gastro-intestinal disturbances, nausea, vomiting, pruritus, rashes, depression of haemopoiesis (*see under* bronchitis).

3. Ampicillin side-effects include urticaria, fever, joint pains, angio-neurotic oedema, anaphylactic shock in hypersensitive patients, diarrhoea, erythematous rashes, or glandular fever (*see under* bronchitis).

4. Nitrofurantoin may cause nausea, vomiting, rashes, peripheral neuropathy, pulmonary infiltration, allergic liver damage.

5. Nalidixic acid may cause a wide variety of side-effects including diarrhoea and vomiting, rashes, fever, arthralgia, and photo-toxicity. It should not be used in pregnancy or lactation, or in patients with impaired renal or hepatic function.

6. The treatments suggested are alternatives, and should cure most infections, and cover most allergic problems in patients.

Enuresis

Treatment

Imipramine   Child dose: Not under 7 years.
                                     7 to 11 years:
                                        25-50 mg:
                                     11 and over 50-75 mg.

Detrusor instability

Treatment

Imipramine   Adult dose: 25 mg three times daily.

Important notes

1. Imipramine may cause dry mouth and other anticholinergic side-effects. Also tachycardia, sweating, and sometimes sleep disturbances in children. (Other side-effects at this dosage are rare.)

Cost

Trimethoprim	100 mg	100 tabs =	£3.05
	200 mg	100 tabs =	£4.50
	50 mg/5 ml suspension	100 ml =	£6.90
Co-trimoxazole	480 mg	100 tabs =	£4.85
	240 mg/5 ml suspension	500 ml =	£9.80
Ampicillin	250 mg	100 caps =	£3.35
	500 mg	100 caps =	£7.00
	125 mg/5 ml suspension	500 ml =	£3.80
	250 mg/5 ml syrup	500 ml =	£6.15
Nitrofurantoin	50 mg	100 tabs =	£1.90
	100 mg	100 tabs =	£13.85
	25 mg/5 ml suspension	500 ml =	£7.50
Nalidixic acid	500 mg	100 tabs =	£10.54
	300 mg/5 ml suspension	500 ml =	£30.00
Imipramine	10 mg	100 tabs =	70p
	25 mg	100 tabs =	65p
	25 mg/5 ml syrup	500 ml =	£9.00

Worms

Treatment

Pripsen OTC (piperazine 4 g sennosides 15.3 mg)

Adult dose: One sachet.
Child dose:
3 months to 1 year: 5 ml granules;
1–6 years: 10 ml;
over 6 years: one sachet.
Repeat all after 14 days.

Mebendazole	Adult dose:	100 mg once only. Repeat after 14 days.
	Child dose:	Over 2 years: 100 mg. Repeat after 14 days.

Important notes

1. Treat whole family and emphasize good hygiene.
2. Beware nail-biters and thumb suckers.
3. Pripsen may cause nausea, vomiting, diarrhoea, urticaria, rarely dizziness, paraesthesia, muscular incoordination.
4. Mebendazole occasionally causes abdominal pain, diarrhoea.
5. Both preparations have been found to be teratogenic in animals and should not be used if pregnancy is a possibility.

Cost

Pripsen sachets	piperazine 4 g sennosides 15.3 mg	2 sachets =	93p
Mebendazole	100 mg	6 tabs	= £1.57
	100 mg/5 ml suspension	30 ml	= £1.82

Appendix

Drug treatments normally initiated by hospital consultants

AIDS/HIV Infection
Treatment

Zidovudine caps	Adult:	200–300 mg 3–4 times daily or 3.5 mg/kg.

Carcinoma of breast

Tamoxifen	10–40 mg twice daily.

Epilepsy

1. Phenobarbitone — 60–180 mg at night.
2. Primidone — 125–500 mg three times daily.
3. Sodium valproate — 100–500 mg three times daily.

Glaucoma

1. Pilocarpine eye-drops — Instil 3–6 times daily.
2. Timolol eye-drops — Instil twice daily.

Manic depression

Lithium carbonate — 250 mg to 2 g daily.

Prophylaxis in pregnancy

Iron and Folic acid — One daily.

Thrombo-embolism/Platelet disorders

1. Warfarin — 3–9 mg daily.
2. Dipyridamole — 100–200 mg three times daily.

Important notes

1. We have not attempted to include all the various insulins, dressings, stoma equipment, etc.
2. Prescribers, although acting on the advice of hospital colleagues, are responsible for the care of their patients.

Cost

Zidovudine	100 mg	100 caps = £114.60
Tamoxifen	100 mg	100 tabs = £25.65
	20 mg	100 tabs = £31.15
Phenobarbitone	30 mg	100 tabs = 65p

Primidone	250 mg	100 tabs =	£1.60
Sodium valproate	200 mg	100 tabs =	£6.60
	500 mg	100 tabs =	£16.45
Pilocarpine eye-drops 0.5%, 1%	10 ml	=	£1.11
Timolol eye-drops	0.25%	5 ml =	£5.18
	0.5%	5 ml =	£5.82
Lithium carbonate	250 mg	100 =	£2.65

Index

ACE inhibitors 29
acne vulgaris 55
acupuncture 38
acyclovir 39, 57
addiction, lorazepam 6
agitation 6
AIDS 59, 71
alcohol, metronidazole 51
allergy 1
allopurinol 8
alpha-blocker 30
Alphosyl 52
aluminium hydroxide 24
amiloride 15
amitriptyline 20
amoxycillin 66
amphotericin 39
ampicillin
  bronchitis 12
  dental abcess 40
  otitis media 66
  sinusitis 64
  urinary infection 68
anaemia 2
anal discomfort 34
anal fissure 34
analgesics 46, 59
angina pectoris 4
anorexia 61
antacids 24
anticoagulants 72
antihistamines 1
Anusol 34
Anusol-HC 34
anxiety 6
aqueous cream 52
arthritis 7
Asilone 24
aspirin
  angina 5
  with codeine 47

migraine 37
myocardial infarction 5
  pain 46
asthma 9
atenolol 29
atrial fibrillation 15

baclofen 43
beclomethasone
  allergy 1
  asthma 10
bendrofluazide
  cardiac failure 14
  hypertension 29
  premenstrual syndrome 49
benserazide
  Madopar 44
benzodiazepines 6
benzoyl peroxide 55
benzyl benzoate 56
beta-blockers 4, 29
Betadine paint 57
betamethasone
  eczema 52
  psoriasis 53
bisacodyl 16
blepharitis 28
breast carcinoma 71
Brevinor 18
bronchitis 12
bulk laxatives 16

calcium antagonist 29
campylobacter enteritis 22
candidiasis
  oral 39
  vaginal 50
captopril 29

Index

carbamazepine
  epilepsy 42
  neuralgia 43
carbidopa
  Sinemet 44
carcinoma of breast 71
cardiac failure 14
cardiac glycoside 15
catarrh 63
cellulitis 54
chlamydia 51
chloramphenicol
  blepharitis 28
  conjunctivitis 28
chlorhexidine 40, 56
chlormethiazole 32
chlorpheniramine 1
chlorpromazine
  agitation 6
  terminal care 61
chlortetracycline 3% cream 54
cimetidine 24
clomipramine 20
clonidine
  menopause 35
  migraine 36
clotrimazole
  tinea 57
  vaginitis 50
co-codamol 47
co-codaprin 47
codeine linctus 64
codeine
  aspirin 47
  paracetamol 47
codeine phosphate 22
  diarrhoea 22
co-dydramol 47
common cold 63
compulsive neurosis 21
confusion 61
conjunctivitis 28
constipation 16, 60
contraception 18
co-proxamol 47
corneal ulcer 28
corticosteroid side-effects 11
co-trimoxazole
  acne 55

bone-marrow depression 13
bronchitis 12
  otitis media 66
cough 64
cramp 48
Crohn's disease 22
cyclizine 60
Cyclo-progynova 35
cytotoxic drug 60

dendritic corneal ulcer 28
dental abcess 40
depression 20
dermatitis 52
detrusor instability 69
dexamethasone 61
diabetes mellitus 26
diamorphine 59
diarrhoea 22, 60
diazepam
  anxiety 6
  spasticity 43
dienoestrol 35
diet
  constipation 17
  diabetes 26
  irritable bowel 33
digoxin 15
dihydrocodeine 47
dimethicone cream 52
dipyridamole 72
Dithrocream 53
diuretics 14, 29
docusate sodium 17
domperidone 60
dothiepin 20
doxycycline 13
dry eyes 28
dry mouth 21
duodenal ulcer 24
Dyazide 15, 29
dydrogesterone 49
dysmenorrhea 49
dyspepsia 24

ear wax 46
eczema

Index

acute 52
  dry 52
emulsifying ointment 52
enalapril 29
endocrine conditions 26
enuresis 69
epilepsy 42
ergotamine 37
erysipelas 55
erythromycin
  acne 55
  bronchitis 13
  diarrhoea 22
  otitis media 66
  sinusitis 64
  throat infection 65
evening primrose, oil of 49
extrapyramidal effects
  metoclopramide 25, 37
  prochlorperazine 41
  tranquillizers 6
eye conditions 28

faecal softeners 17
ferrous gluconate 3
ferrous sulphate 2
flucloxacillin
  cellulitis 54
  impetigo 54
folic acid 3
frusemide 15
furunculosis 56

gardnerella vaginitis 51
gastric ulcer 24
Gaviscon 24
glaucoma 72
glibenclamide 26
glycerin thymol mouth wash 61
glycerol suppositories 17
glyceryl trinitrate 4
gout 8

haloperidol 60
hayfever 1

herpes
  labialis 39
  simplex 57
  stomatitis 39
  zoster 57
hiatus hernia 25
HIV 71
hormone replacement therapy 35
hydrocortisone
  mouth ulcer 38
  Nystaform-HC 52
  skin conditions 52
hydroxocobalamin 3
hyoscine hydrobromide 62
hypertension 29
hypnotics 32
hypothyroidism 27
hypromellose drops 28

ibuprofen 7
ichthyosis 52
idoxuridine
  corneal ulcer 28
  herpes zoster 57
  oral herpes 39
imipramine
  depression 20
  detrusor instability 69
  enuresis 69
impetigo 54
indomethacin
  arthritis 8
  gout 8
  metastases 59
inflammatory bowel disease 22
insomnia 32
intracranial pressure, raised 61
iron and folic acid 72
irritable bowel syndrome 33
isosorbide dinitrate 4
isosorbide mononitrate 4
ispaghula husk 16

lactic acidosis 26
lactulose 17

Index

laxatives
  bulk 16
  osmotic 17
  stimulant 16
levodopa
  Madopar 44
  Sinemet 44
levonorgestrel in Cycloprogynova 35
lignocaine
  gel 34
  injection 8
linctus
  codeine 64
  simplex 64
lindane 56
lithium carbonate 72
Locorten-vioform 45
Logynon 18
Loperamide 22
lorazepam 6

Maalox 24
Madopar 44
magnesium trisilicate 24
manic depression 72
Marvelon 18
mebendazole 71
mebeverine 33
mefenamic acid 49
menopause 35
metformin 26
methyldopa 30
methyl prednisolone 8
metoclopramide
  dyspepsia 25
  migraine 37
metoprolol
  angina 4
  hypertension 29
metronidazole
  dental abscess 40
  vaginal discharge 51
mianserin 20
Microgynon 30 18
Micronor 19
migraine 36
morning-after pill 19
morphine 59

mouth dry 61
mouth infections 38, 61
mouth ulcers 38
myocardial infarction 5

nalidixic acid 68
nappy rash 52
naproxen
  arthritis 8
  gout 8
nausea 41, 59
Neogest 19
neuralgia 43
  post-herpetic 43
neurological disorders 42
nifedepine
  angina 4
  hypertension 29
nitrates 4
nitrazepam 32
nitrofurantoin 68
non-steroidal anti-inflammatory
    drugs 7, 8, 59
norethisterone 49
Nuelin 11
Nystaform-HC 52
nystatin
  Nystaform-HC 52
  oral candida 39
  pruritus vulvae 50

obsessive neuroses 21
oesophagitis 24
oestradiol
  Cycloprogynova 35
oestrogen therapy 35
oilatum 52
olive oil 46
oral candida 39
oral herpes 39
oral hygiene 40
orphenadrine 44
osmotic laxatives 17
otitis media 66
otitis externa 45
Otosporin 45
overdose, dextropropoxyphene 47

Index

Ovran 19
Ovranette 18
Ovysmen 18
oxytetracycline
  acne 55
  bronchitis 12

pain 46, 59
paracetamol 46
  with codeine 47
  with dihydrocodeine 47
  migraine 37
  throat infections 65
parkinsonism 44
penicillin
  cellulitis 54
  dental abscess 40
  erysipelas 55
  throat infection 65
peptic ulcer 24
pethidine 47
phenobarbitone 72
phenothiazines
  agitation 6
  parkinsonism 44
phenytoin, epilepsy 42
pilocarpine 72
piroxicam 8
pizotifen 37
Polytar 53
potassium chloride 15
prazosin 30
prednisolone 61
  enema 22
Premarin 35
premenstrual syndrome 49
primidone 72
Pripsen 70
prochlorperazine 41
promethazine 32
propranolol
  angina 4
  anxiety 6
  hypertension 29
  migraine 37
pruritus vulvae 50
pseudoephedrine 63
psoriasis 52

pyridoxine 49

quinine sulphate 48

raised intracranial pressure 61
ranitidine 24
respiratory symptoms 62
restlessness 61

salbutamol 9
salicylic acid collodion 58
scabies 56
senna 16
simple linctus 64
Sinemet 44
sinusitis 64
skin conditions 52
skin infections 54
sodium chloride and glucose 22
sodium citrate enema 60
sodium cromoglycate allergy 1
  asthma 10
sodium valproate 72
spasticity 42
spironolactone 15
steam inhalations 63
stimulant laxatives 16
sulphasalazine 22
syringe pump 59

tamoxifen 71
temazepam 32
tennis elbow 8
terbutaline 10
terfenadine 1
terminal care 59
tetracyclic drug 20
theophylline 10
thioridazine 6
throat infections 65
thrombo-embolism 72
thymol glycerin mouthwash 61
thyroxine 27
timolol 72
tinea 57

Index

tolbutamide 26
trichomonal infection 51
tricyclic drugs 20
trimeprazine 32
trimethoprim 12, 68
trinitrate, glyceryl 4
Trinordiol 18

ulcerative colitis 23
upper respiratory tract infections 63
urinary tract conditions 68
urinary tract infection 68
urticaria 1

vaginal discharge 50

valproate, sodium 72
vertigo 41
vitamin B_{12} deficiency 3
vomiting 41, 59

warfarin 72
warts 57
wax, ear 46
Whitfield's ointment 57
worms 70

zidovudine 71
zinc cream 52